Nursing Models and Nursing Practice

Second Edition

Peter Aggleton and Helen Chalmers

palgrave

First edition published as *Nursing Models and the Nursing Process* 1986
Reprinted eleven times
Second edition 2000

Published by
PALGRAVE
Houndmills, Basingstoke, Hampshire RG21 6XS and
175 Fifth Avenue, New York, N.Y. 10010
Companies and representatives throughout the world

PALGRAVE is the new global academic imprint of
St. Martin's Press LLC Scholarly and Reference Division and
Palgrave Publishers Ltd (formerly Macmillan Press Ltd).

ISBN–13: 978–0–333–48822–5
ISBN–10: 0–333–48822–9

This book is printed on paper suitable for recycling and made from fully managed and sustained forest sources.

A catalogue record for this book is available from the British Library.

11 10   9   8   7
09 08 07 06 05

Editing and origination by
Aardvark Editorial, Mendham, Suffolk

Printed and bound in Great Britain b
Creative Print & Design (Wales), Ebb

Contents

Acknowledgements

We would like to thank the *Nursing Times* for permission to reproduce elements of the following articles in Chapters 9–11 of this book: P. J. Aggleton and H. Chalmers (1989) Neuman's systems model, *Nursing Times*, 85, 51, 27–9; P. J. Aggleton and H. Chalmers (1990) King's model, *Nursing Times*, 86, 1, 38–9; P. J. Aggleton and H. Chalmers (1990) Peplau's development model, *Nursing Times*, 86, 2, 38–40; and I. M. King (1981) *A Theory for Nursing: Systems, Concepts, Process*, John Wiley & Sons, New York, p. 11.

Every effort has been made to trace all the copyright holders but if any have been inadvertently overlooked the publishers will be pleased to make the necessary arrangements at the first opportunity.

The reader should note that all references in this book to one gender should also be read as applying to the other gender unless specifically indicated otherwise.

Preface

When the first edition of this book, *Nursing Models and the Nursing Process*, was written in the mid-1980s, terms such as 'nursing process', 'nursing models' and 'nursing theory' were relatively new, at least to many nurses in Britain. While some nurses were initially suspicious of what they saw as the introduction of more jargon into nursing, a more sober assessment of the contribution of nursing models and the nursing process to patient care has become possible as time has passed. It is now widely recognised that, when appropriately used, nursing models help to focus the nursing role, assist in individualising care and provide a guide to practice. They allow nurses to communicate with one another about what they are doing and may, in time, facilitate the emergence of nursing theory – as a unique body of knowledge central to nursing's emergence as a fully fledged profession.

Until relatively recently, nursing has made few claims to having a body of knowledge of its own. Instead, it has seemingly been content to 'borrow' understandings from the natural, medical and social sciences – from biology and biochemistry, from anatomy and physiology and, more recently, from psychology and sociology. While these kinds of knowledge can be helpful when providing care, there are other sources of insight that can also be drawn upon. These include ethical knowledge, the moral principles that define nurses' accountability to patients and to each other; aesthetic knowledge, linked to creativity, sensitivity and empathy; and personal knowledge derived from reflection on past experience (Chinn and Kramer, 1995). Together with scientific knowledge, these other ways of understanding establish the unique perspective on people and health that nursing offers.

New terminology and new ways of thinking about issues are constantly being introduced in nursing, as in other walks of life. Some of the consequences of this may be useful in that they may help nurses to think about their experiences more precisely or in different ways. Others may be less so, particularly if they discourage nurses from thinking critically about the care they give. Additionally, the introduction of new ideas and techniques into nursing practice can lead to the development of a better understanding of people and their health-related needs. It may cause us to question some of the taken-for-granted assumptions that we may have about how best to care for patients, and about the relative responsibilities of nurses, doctors, friends and relatives in the caring process.

Over the past decade, there has been an opportunity to reflect on these different viewpoints and on the ways in which nursing has changed to meet changing circumstances. In many parts of the world, there have been dramatic changes in health service organisation, in the roles and responsibilities of different kinds of health care workers, and in public expectations about what might be expected of health services, be they provided by the state or the private sector. These changes have been accompanied by innovations in nurse education, nurse management and the planning and delivery of nursing care. We will begin, therefore, by examining some of these changes and the opportunities and challenges they pose for nursing today. Having set the scene in this way, we will define some of the key concepts and terms that will be used throughout this book before describing in detail some of the most important models of nursing and their application to nursing care.

In preparing this book, we owe an immense debt to our friends, families and colleagues for their support and understanding. We are also grateful to the many nurses whom we have taught over the years, who have challenged us with their questions and responses to the various models described here, and whose insight has been valuable in offering an evaluation of different approaches to care. We would also like to thank our various publishers and editors at Palgrave, but most particularly Richenda Milton-Thompson for her faith in this project and for encouraging us to see it through to its proper conclusion.

PETER AGGLETON and HELEN CHALMERS
Brighton and Bath, 1999

Reference

Chinn, P. L. and Kramer, M. K. (1995) *Theory and Nursing: A Systematic Approach*. St Louis, C.V. Mosby.

Chapter 1 Nursing models in a changing context

The health context in which nurses work has changed enormously since nursing models were first explored in relation to clinical practice in the UK and other European countries. Many aspects of nursing practice and the role of the nurse have also changed. What remains, however, is the need for a knowledge base concerning the nature of people and their health-related needs from which nurses can develop their clinical practice. Nursing models continue to provide this knowledge base. Understandings about the nature of people and the nature of health will always be central to care even if such understandings are not always called nursing models.

Without knowledge about the nature of people and their health-related needs, nurses would be unable to go about their work in anything but a haphazard way. In addition, nurses working together should ideally practise with shared understandings about people (that is, with the same model of nursing) to ensure continuity of appropriate nursing care. What has changed over the past two decades is many nurses' familiarity in working with a model of nursing, although to date it is fair to say that most nurses' experience is limited to just one or two models. It is therefore timely to revisit what models have to offer.

In setting the scene for a further exploration of how nursing models can contribute to the practice and development of nursing, we will necessarily have to be selective and somewhat brief. The many changes that have occurred and continue to occur in the management of health care and in nursing are well described in a variety of other texts (see, for example, Gabe *et al.*, 1991; Jolley and Brykczynska, 1993; Hunt and Wainwright, 1994; Davies, 1995; Mohan 1995; Klein, 1995). What we offer here is an overview of some of the key changes that have had an impact on nurses and nursing. The overview has two parts. The first examines the changing context of health care delivery, including public expectations of the service provided. The second looks at the current role of the nurse, including changes in nurse education and growing professionalisation. While such a division is in many ways arbitrary, it is possible, by identifying those changes which impinge more directly on nurses, to understand the contribution that nursing models can make to the situations in which nurses find themselves.

Health care delivery

Following the publication of the White Paper *Working for Patients* (Secretary of State for Health, 1989) and subsequent legislation in 1990, many changes have occurred in the UK National Health Service (NHS) and in the independent sector. The introduction of the internal market in the NHS, for example, brought the notion of competition in health care provision into sharp focus, with NHS Trusts and the independent sector competing for service agreements.

The professed aim of these changes was to improve standards of care for patients, but Mohan (1995), among many others, has taken issue with this. He believes that three main objectives lay behind such moves: to restructure the welfare state, to impose greater managerial control, and to pander to certain key groups of Conservative government supporters. Complex administrative systems, coupled with pressure for more and more so-called efficiency savings, caused concern among many health care workers, including nurses. The commitment to money following patients made short-term, acute care a more attractive management option because it was seen as potentially much more lucrative. The traditional 'Cinderella' services, such as the care of those with learning difficulties and the care of elderly people, were therefore increasingly at risk, as evidenced by the transfer of responsibility for them out of the health service.

Media attention to the negative consequences of this changed structure of health service provision for, for example, mentally ill or elderly people failing to obtain adequate community care revealed but the tip of the iceberg for those most in need of long-term support and care. A health service that increasingly revolves around acute care provision marginalises those most affected by health and social problems linked to disability, old age, unemployment and social and economic deprivation. For these people, the previous government's concern to place responsibility for health and well-being increasingly on the individual seemed especially inept. As has been repeatedly demonstrated over many years (see, for example, DoH, 1998a; Townsend *et al.*, 1988), the social divisions in health remain largely unchanged in our society. Changes to the structure and management of the NHS are unlikely to have a positive impact on wider health and social problems. Indeed, by concentrating on acute services and by encouraging a two-tier health service, in part through GP fund-holding, the previous government's so-called reforms threatened the most vulnerable. The burden of care in many cases thus fell on individuals and on their families or friends, many of whom were ill equipped in terms of skills and resources to meet the care demand.

Such concerns have led to a major re-evaluation of the wisdom of caring for some client groups in the community with little hospital back-up when severe problems occur. However, some mental health nurses in particular may find the philosophy or model they currently work with at odds with government demands for the enforcement of medication regimes. Changes are also underway to alter the system of GP fund-holding and to create several forms of Primary Care Group so that there is less overt competition between individual practices and local health care Trusts. It also seems probable that nurses will have more input into decisions made in Primary Care Groups than they did with GP fund-holding.

Given the previous government's interest in acute care, it is not surprising that methods of demonstrating the effectiveness of health care provision increasingly seek to confirm that the health service is providing more acute services for less money. Government attention to waiting list figures is a typical example of this trend. If the criteria for inclusion on a waiting list are appropriately chosen, it is not difficult to show, in the short term at least, that more patients are waiting less time for surgery to take place. Ignored by such figures are those excluded from the waiting list, those who remove themselves from the list through either death or spontaneous recovery, and the quality of the care received once someone moves from the list and into a service setting.

Pressure to see outpatients within a specified maximum time encourages short, often inadequate consultations with doctors and nurses, coupled with potential poor patient satisfaction and compliance with the information given. District nurses have been subject to similar stresses to ensure adherence to appointment times. Such concerns, while they may improve the service for a few people, fail to take account of the nature of much health care, in which the amount of time required to give quality care may be difficult to determine in advance. For many nurses, it is this apparent lack of understanding demonstrated by managers that

3

causes further disquiet. To challenge such limited ways of evaluating the service, nurses must be able to identify alternative methods that can be supported by a sound knowledge base. These include the use of carefully evaluated nursing models.

The government initiative to set out citizens' rights and expectations in relation to service industries has taken the form of the *Patient's Charter* (DoH, 1995) in the health service. The Charter identifies certain rights and standards, one of which relates to the expectation that a named nurse, midwife or health visitor will be responsible for each patient. In most clinical areas, nurses have therefore introduced the concept of the named nurse. Broadly welcomed by many nurses, the concept has in some areas been closely allied to primary nursing. In others, it is more limited in scope and involves the identification of a named nurse for only a short duration of care, sometimes just one worked shift. Unfortunately, such variations are often a reflection of constraints within health care provision rather than the result of well-thought-through nursing decisions. In particular, staff shortages and inadequate resources have threatened the introduction and the effectiveness of the named nurse role.

The Charter also stresses people's right to receive health care on the basis of clinical need and the right to clear information about any proposed treatments so that decisions can be made about the choices available. Nursing models have always paid greater attention to the patient's role in decision-making than has the medical model, and as such they provide a useful basis for the development of the nurse's role as patient advocate. Being an advocate may involve supplying relevant information to patients about treatment options and supporting patients to make difficult decisions. Through the nature of nursing work, it is frequently the nurse who is able to discuss options and possibilities with a patient at a time when the patient feels ready for such a discussion.

Linked to information-giving and decision-making is the importance of consent to treatment. The traditional emphasis on written consent obtained before operative procedures has developed to include an acknowledgement of the importance of implied consent, through the actions of a patient prior to a more limited procedure, and of verbal consent following discussion about some intervention strategies. Patient involvement in goal-setting and care planning is a feature of most nursing models and provides an important way of establishing a patient's agreement to planned care. There are other recent innovations in the ways in which people can make their wishes known. Advance directives, or living wills, are drawn up by some people to indicate in advance their wishes about treatment options. Such documents are currently not legally binding, but the United Kingdom Central Council for Nursing, Midwifery and Health Visiting (UKCC, 1996) has advised that such expressed wishes should be respected by nurses.

In the *Health of the Nation*, five key areas were identified in each of which improvement in health status was made a priority (DoH, 1992). This strategic plan focused attention and resources onto these identified areas in an effort to meet set targets. Government recognition that maintaining and improving health is a crucial aspect of care was long overdue, but a worrying emphasis on individual lifestyles and individual responsibility pervaded much *Health of the Nation* literature, with a scant acknowledgement of the role of social structure and social inequality. A subsequent evaluation of the *Health of the Nation* strategy has shown this approach to be flawed both conceptually and with respect to implementation. There was little evidence that the *Health of the Nation* changed the perspectives and behaviours of health authorities, and despite a rhetorical commitment to healthy alliances, a lack of cross-departmental commitment and ownership set serious limits on what could be achieved (Stationery Office, 1998a).

The government has subsequently sought to promote a more expanded response to health and the remedying of health inequalities. The White Paper *Saving Lives: Our Healthier Nation* emphasises the value of cross-departmental working and greater 'partnership' between local authorities, health authorities, the private sector and the voluntary sector (DoH, 1999). The establishment of Health Improvement Programmes, the designation of Health Action Zones and the continued encouragement for joint working between health and social services (see, for example, DoH, 1998b) has also sought to operationalise some of these commitments. The challenges are substantial, however, since, as the Independent Inquiry into Inequalities in Health recently showed, there remain substantial gaps between the health of the rich and that of the poor (Stationery Office, 1998b). Providing equitably and appropriately for those who are marginalised and socially excluded from mainstream society is likely to remain a challenge for the forseeable future.

Nurses have an important contribution to make in trying to meet targets for health, both through their contact with individuals and through their understanding of the wider social issues impinging on health chances. Nursing models all go beyond the individual explanations for ill-health that have been so criticised of late, and many offer useful insights into the interplay between individual lifestyles and personal and social circumstances. They thus afford nurses appropriate frameworks around which to plan health promotion interventions.

Nursing role

A casual visitor to a hospital or other health care setting might think that little has changed for nurses over the past decade. The majority of nurses still wear a traditional and recognisable uniform, and are to be found in areas where care is provided or advice offered to patients, their relatives and their friends. However, behind this seemingly unchanged exterior, much has altered. In particular, nurses are now educated through a different system of training. They are educated to a higher academic level, and the work they do and the way in which they do it have, in many areas of health care, changed considerably.

With the introduction of Project 2000 (P2K) came not only a different system of initial education and training, but also a commitment to the development of a more knowledgeable practitioner prepared for the demands of nursing in the year 2000 and beyond. The analysis, evaluation and application of models of nursing thus became integral to the new curriculum in many colleges of nursing, largely because models were recognised as being one major step towards the development of a unique body of nursing knowledge, as opposed to that associated with medicine. This is not to say that nurses are now entirely comfortable with the notion that patient care can be improved by using a recognised model of nursing. Indeed, for many nurses, the process of introducing a nursing model into clincal practice has been complicated by other issues, such as the way in which nursing could be organised in a particular setting and concerns about the scope of professional practice.

However, raising the academic level (students now gain a nursing qualification and a higher education diploma at least) has meant that P2K students have the necessary skills to assess the potential value of nursing models to practice and to contribute to their use and evaluation. It remains too early fully to evaluate the impact of P2K on nursing practice and nurses' professionalisation, although concern has been expressed about the reduced amount of patient/client contact that students have, and the continuing unwillingness of both managers and most doctors to recognise nursing as a profession (Casey, 1996).

P2K students also undertake their training in colleges of nursing that form part of the British system of higher education. This can mean that nursing students have more opportunities to mix with other undergraduates and to benefit from dialogue with, and study alongside, people with different interests and expertise. The mutual advantage that this should bring in terms of understanding the wider context of health care and how individuals regard health issues is difficult to evaluate. It is arguably an ideal preparation for being open and receptive to some of the concepts addressed within nursing models.

When the first edition of this text was published, there was considerable criticism from some nurses that many of the ideas were American in origin. At the time, many practising nurses felt understandably more drawn to the ideas expressed in models that were closer to the medical model with which they were familiar. Such models include the Roper, Logan and Tierney model and those developed by Virginia Henderson and Dorothea Orem. More than a decade later, we believe that greater familiarity with these models and how they can benefit patient and client care has encouraged nurses to select other, often more challenging, models for application and evaluation. In this context, American models of nursing still have much to offer, especially as the development of new models in Britain has seen few models offering a real challenge to the medical model.

Post-registration nurse education has also undergone many changes. There is an increasing demand for courses leading to degree status. In England, this has been linked to the Framework for Post-Registration Studies established by the English National Board for Nursing, Midwifery and Health Visiting (ENB, 1991). As with P2K, the Framework emphasises the need for education to be closely linked to the practice of nursing. The academic acknowledgement of a development of knowledge and skill therefore goes hand in hand with professional recognition. Thus, the ENB initiative has been important in highlighting the need for nurses' further study to be closely linked to the contribution that a greater understanding can make to patient care.

Models of nursing have the potential to provide a unifying force for the study of many disciplines that can inform practice. This potential has so far been poorly developed, subjects such as psychology, physiology and alternative therapies often being taught as discrete topics and applied to patient problems generated through a medicalised approach to care. Through the study of models, understandings from other disciplines can be subjected to more rigorous evaluation because they frequently form the theoretical underpinning of the model itself and thereby hold the potential to challenge rather than just broaden the understandings gained from medicine.

A related and significant change for nurses has been the requirement for them to maintain a personal professional portfolio as part of the Post-Registration Education and Practice (PREP) requirements developed by the UKCC. The putting together of a profile is seen as a way of encouraging nurses to reflect on their current knowledge and skills by reviewing their past experience and identifying the learning that has taken place. As with the Framework, there is a clear emphasis on the importance of practical experience to the development of a knowledge base that is unique to nursing. Nurses compiling their profile are encouraged to be self-assessors so that they gain the ability to recognise their own achievements as well as identify aspects of their practice and knowledge that could be further developed.

For many nurses, the requirement to construct a profile offers an ideal opportunity to reflect on the learning associated with the use of models in practice and a chance to consider how models could be used to further enhance the provision of high-quality care. For a few nurses, this has led them to formulate their own model of care, but it has more often provided the stimulus to consider the contribution that different models can make to patient care. Because it is likely that many nurses have worked in a meaningful way with only a few models of nursing, it is hoped that this second edition of *Nursing Models and Nursing Practice* will assist those nurses who now practise confidently with one or two models to revisit and explore others that have the potential to help them develop their practice further.

The role and scope of practice have also changed significantly. Where once the range of skills seen as appropriate for the qualified nurse was fairly tightly controlled and any development was seen as 'extending' the role, requiring agreement and assessment by someone in a senior and often medical position, nurses are now encouraged to develop their role in diverse ways. Such developments are regarded by many as the best way for nurses to fulfil their obligations to the people for whom they care. (For example, nurses may develop the skill of setting up an intravenous infusion because they feel that this is an appropriate nursing role in their clinical area.) However, there is for many nurses considerable conflict in deciding whether or not to extend the scope of practice in this way, given that those activities and commitments central to nursing may then be in jeopardy through lack of nursing time. Some nurses are encouraged by those in management positions to take on tasks traditionally seen as lying within the medical domain, often to help to avoid the shortfall in medical hours caused by the reduction in time worked by junior doctors.

A few nurses continue to see medical knowledge and tasks as being in some way superior to nursing and may develop new skills accordingly. Fatchett (1994) has argued that this view of the superiority of medical knowledge on the part of some nurses helps to explain why nursing has failed to achieve its own knowledge base and accompanying professional status. Such an argument may also explain the continuing reluctance of some nurses to do more than pay lip service to the value of nursing models to practice. It is not uncommon for nurses in a clinical area to have selected a particular model for use and yet struggle with the changes to practice that it advocates. Until nurses themselves value the unique contribution that they make to health care and the special body of knowledge that informs their practice, the subordinate role adopted by many nurses to that undertaken by doctors will continue. This poses many threats to the achievement of high-quality care, not least because it may deter nurses from establishing an equal role with doctors in their discussions about planning patient care. Such a lack of equity ill equips nurses to act effectively as the patient's advocate or to justify nursing interventions that stem from particular nursing models and other sources of nursing knowledge, for example research studies.

Progress towards greater equality and professionalisation can be achieved in a variety of ways, including nurses gaining degree-level qualifications, developing their understanding of the uniqueness of nursing, exploring the value of clinical supervision and carrying out research to provide evidence for particular nursing strategies. Many of these developments hinge on the study and use of nursing models in practice. Models provide theoretical frameworks from which further understanding about people and their health-related needs can develop, and from which nursing strategies can be justified and their effectiveness evaluated. The current emphasis on evidence-based practice and clinical effectiveness is one that is welcomed by all the nursing theorists featured in the following chapters.

While some nurses may feel that a model of nursing is a fixed set of ideas about people and their health-related needs, many nurses now recognise the enormous opportunity for further research that an increased understanding of models offers. Whereas, when the first edition of this book was written, there was a tendency to implement a selected model rather rigidly, there is now more confidence to work creatively and questioningly with the ideas embodied in a particular model.

The Department of Health (DoH, 1993) advocated the introduction of clinical supervision in 1993, although Jones (1998) argues that it is still in its infancy in many areas of nursing practice. A key element of clinical supervision involves asking questions about what has taken place and why. Part of this should involve a consideration of the contribution made by the particular understandings of people and the nurse–patient relationship put forward by the nursing model used. More recently, an information pack has been produced for nurses, midwives and health visitors to enable them to evaluate their clinical effectiveness (NHS Executive, 1998), encouraging them to use the available literature to become more aware of what other nurses have done. This can include reference to the original work of nursing theorists and evaluations of the appropriateness of their models to practice in particular areas.

The role of the nurse has changed more in some practice settings than in others. For example, the supernumerary status of nursing students throughout much of their training has meant that qualified nurses in recognised teaching areas may work with a team of other qualified nurses and unqualified assistants not pursuing a nursing qualification. Thus, some caring personnel working under the supervision of trained nurses have a range of skills rather different from those of the traditional student nurse. Such situations have highlighted the importance of the decisions made by qualified nurses concerning the matching of skills to the demands of patient care, and have sometimes raised concerns about accountability.

The way in which such crucial decisions can be handled with confidence is to base them on reliable information about the patient and on reliable knowledge of the skills of those helping in the delivery of care. Thus, careful and appropriate patient assessment by a qualified nurse has gained even more importance. It is not possible to assess a patient without a set of ideas about people and their health-related needs. At no time should, or indeed could, a nurse ask questions about everything to do with a patient or client. This would be both intrusive and largely irrelevant. What is crucial is that a nurse finds out about those things which are pertinent to the person's health status; this involves considerable selectivity, which must be based on knowledge rather than intuition.

The use of an appropriate nursing model informs assessment by establishing the kind of information required, the detail that is likely to be helpful and the ways in which the information might best be gathered. The chapters that follow provide examples of a variety of assessments and of how assessment techniques can differ. Crucially, the examples offered all develop from understandings inherent in the model in use rather than from a particular nurse's view of health and illness. It is essential that nurses working together, as primary or associate nurses or in discrete teams, should practise with a shared understanding about the people for whom they care. Without this shared vision of what is to be achieved, there may be omissions of important information during assessment, or the inclusion of irrelevancies. Only after detailed assessment and planning is the qualified nurse in a position to delegate certain aspects of patient care to others.

A model can also help to determine the kinds of intervention best suited to the patient's needs and can thus contribute to the decision of who should intervene and in what way. In this way, decisions informed by the thoughtful application of a recognised nursing model can go a long way towards meeting the demands of accountability. As indicated in the UKCC *Guidelines for Professional Practice*:

If you delegate work to someone who is not registered with the UKCC, your accountability is to make sure that the person who does the work is able to do it and that appropriate levels of supervision or support are in place. (UKCC, 1996: 9)

The chapters that follow explore some of these concerns surrounding the practice of nursing in relation to particular examples of nursing care. All the examples offered derive from experience in working with genuine patients or potential patients. We hope that you will find them helpful in identifying some of the strengths of nursing models and some of the contexts in which they can be used.

References

Casey, G. (1996) The curriculum revolution and project 2000: a critical evaluation. *Nurse Education Today*, **16**(2): 115–20.

Davies, C. (1995) *Gender and the Professional Predicament in Nursing*. Buckingham, Open University Press.

Department of Health (1992) *Health of the Nation*. London, HMSO.

Department of Health (1993) *A Vision for the Future: The Nursing, Midwifery and Health Visiting Contribution to Health and Health Care*. London, HMSO.

Department of Health (1995) *The Patient's Charter*. London, DoH.

Department of Health (1998) *Partnership in Action: New Opportunities for Joint Working Between Health and Social Services*. London, DoH.

Department of Health (1999) *Saving Lives: Our Healthier Nation*. London, Stationery Office.

English National Board for Nursing, Midwifery and Health Visiting (1991) *Framework for Continuing Professional Education for Nurses, Midwives and Health Visitors: A Guide to Implementation*. London, ENB.

Fatchett, A. (1994) *Politics, Policy and Nursing*. London, Baillière Tindall.

Gabe, J., Calnan, M. and Bury, M. (eds) (1991) *The Sociology of the Health Service*. London, Routledge.

Hunt, G. and Wainwright, P. (eds) (1994) *Expanding the Role of the Nurse: The Scope of Professional Practice*. Oxford, Blackwell Science.

Jolley, M. and Brykczynska, G. (1993) *Nursing: Its Hidden Agendas*. London, Edward Arnold.

Jones, A. (1998) 'Out of the sighs' – an existential-phenomenological method of clinical supervision: the contribution to palliative care. *Journal of Advanced Nursing*, **27**(5): 905–13.

Klein, R. (1995) *The New Politics of the NHS*. London, Longman.

Mohan, J. (1995) *A National Health Service?* Basingstoke, Macmillan.

NHS Executive (1998) *Achieving Effective Practice: A Clinical Effectiveness and Research Information Pack for Nurses, Midwives and Health Visitors*. London, DoH.

Secretary of State for Health (1989) *Working for Patients*. London, HMSO.

Stationery Office (1998a) *Health of the Nation – A Policy Assessed*. London, Stationery Office.

Stationery Office (1998b) *Report of the Independent Inquiry into Inequalities in Health*. London, Stationery Office.

Townsend, P., Davidson, N. and Whitehead, M. (1988) *Inequalities in Health (The Black Report) and the Health Divide*. Harmondsworth, Penguin.

United Kingdom Central Council for Nursing, Midwifery and Health Visiting (1996) *Guidelines for Professional Practice*. London, UKCC.

Chapter 2 Some key concepts

Before looking in detail at a number of different approaches to planning and delivering nursing care, it is helpful to explain certain phrases. In particular, it is important to define what is meant by the terms 'nursing process', 'nursing models' and 'nursing theory', since an understanding of these is vital to what follows.

The nursing process

Until relatively recently, many nurses believed that nursing is best carried out when based on instinct, intuition and empathy, elements that make up the 'calling' that many experience when first attracted to the profession. Such an approach to the planning and delivery of nursing care, alongside a form of apprenticeship training that involved practising acts such as aseptic technique, has since come in for considerable criticism. In 1963, Bonney and Rothberg were among the first to call for a more *systematic* approach to care tailored to the needs of individuals, with attention being paid to the physical, psychological and behavioural aspects of the person. Kelly (1966) extended such ideas to include a focus on social history and cultural background as well as environmental factors affecting health and well-being.

While nurse writers such as these were concerned to broaden the scope of nursing away from intuition and ritual, it was not until 1967, with the publication of Yura and Walsh's book *The Nursing Process* that a discrete number of stages in nursing care were distinguished. Yura and Walsh argued that nursing could, or should, be likened to a problem-solving process in which nurse and patient:

1. together identify the causes of problems requiring intervention
2. make plans to remedy these problems
3. take the necessary steps to alleviate them, and then
4. reflect on what has happened.

The four stages involved in this process, the *nursing process* as Yura and Walsh call it, are assessment, planning, implementation and evaluation. Writers such as Little and Carnevali (1971), Mayers (1972), Crow (1977) and Marriner (1979) have subsequently spelled out in more detail what each of these four original stages involves. More recently, Christenson and Kenney (1990, 1995), Oermann (1991), Wilkinson (1992) and Linberg *et al.* (1994) have found it helpful to distinguish a fifth stage – nursing diagnosis – intermediate between assessment and planning.

Assessment and nursing diagnosis

By placing an emphasis on *assessment*, the nursing process encourages the nurse to identify with the patient potential and actual health problems. While some of these problems may be linked to specific medical conditions, others will be specific to individuals, their psychology and their social and cultural status. Assessment is more often than not a multistage process in which initial ideas are formed about existing health problems, followed by efforts to confirm the existence of these problems and to identify their probable causes.

Nursing diagnosis involves making 'a decisive statement concerning the client's nursing needs' (George, 1995: 21). It differs from medical diagnosis in that it places an emphasis on 'the whole unique person who is interacting with the environment and whose health state – not just the illness or disease – requires nursing intervention' (Christenson and Kenney, 1995: 10).

Planning

By arguing that nursing care should be *planned*, the nursing process encourages the nurse and the person being cared for to set goals. These goals may be short term, intermediate or long term in nature, specifying behaviours that the person receiving care should be able to achieve at the end of given periods of time. Subsequent to goal-setting, decisions must be made about the priority with which each will be tackled and about the techniques that nurses will use in order to achieve each of them. Prioritised goals, along with a statement of the nursing and other actions that need to be taken to achieve them, make up a key part of the care plan.

Intervention

Having specified goals, nurses should be in a position to implement the plan of care by making interventions. Nursing interventions take the form of a series of activities with which nurses are involved in order to help patients to achieve goals. Some authors (for example Kratz, 1979) call these activities 'nursing actions'. Nursing actions can include doing, recording and delegating (Wilkinson, 1992). They can be hygienic, assertive, rehabilitative, supportive, preventive, educative and observational in nature (Campbell, 1980).

Evaluation

By emphasising the importance of evaluation in nursing, the nursing process encourages nurses to compare the actual behaviours of which people are capable at particular points in their care with the goals previously set. Ongoing evaluation of this kind is sometimes called *formative evaluation* since it enables nurses to monitor the effectiveness of their interventions in meeting health-related needs. Formative evaluation is different from *summative evaluation*, which should take place after a nurse has ceased to be involved in the care of an individual.

Both formative and summative evaluation are often concerned with an examination of whether or not goals and objectives have been met, focusing on the *outcomes* associated with particular interventions. Nurses, however, may also be interested in the *processes* by which these outcomes were achieved, the way in which things were done, the person's reaction to them and the manner in which goals were perhaps redefined throughout the time that care was given.

While a number of discrete stages can be identified in the nursing process, it would be wrong to suppose that these take place independently of one another. In reality, there is a cyclical movement from one stage to that which follows as the successful completion of each step provides useful information for the next.

Throughout the chapters that follow, a systematic approach to the delivery of nursing care will be used to demonstrate examples of how a particular model might be used in practice. This systematic approach will most commonly comprise the four stages of the nursing process. However, some nursing theorists have recommended modifications to the process or have suggested a sequence of stages rather different from those of the nursing process. Where this is so, we shall follow the approach advocated for a particular model while at the same time identifying the ways in which it is similar to, and different from, the nursing process.

Nursing models

As we have seen, the nursing process offers a systematic approach to care, one very different both from the routines and task-driven procedures of the past, and from approaches to care that rely solely upon the intuition of the practitioner. By itself, however, the nursing process is a somewhat empty approach. It exhorts nurses to assess but does not tell them what to look for; it advocates planning yet says little about the form that care plans should take. It talks of intervention yet fails to specify what might be appropriate interventions in particular circumstances, and it calls for evaluation without specifying the standards against which comparisons should be made. In order to make the nursing process work, we need a further set of ideas about people and the factors that can cause health-related problems to arise, a framework, if you like, with which to activate the nursing process and bring it to life. This is where models of nursing have relevance.

In general terms, a model of something is a way of representing it – a device that attempts to explain something and by so doing facilitates a better understanding. Many models are physical and can be touched, taken apart and put back together again. Plastic models of the eye and ear, or of the organs within the abdominal cavity, are examples of this kind of representation. Other models are more abstract. They cannot be touched or taken apart, but they may be looked at or thought about. Diagrams showing the interrelated processes at work in digestion or respiration are examples of this latter kind of representation.

In nursing, too, there are abstract models of what nursing is or *should* be about. Their aim is to help those who use them to understand more fully what they are doing and why they are doing it. These models tell us about the nature of people, the kinds of thing that can cause health problems, what nurses should look for when carrying out an assessment, how to plan, what kinds of intervention are appropriate and so on. Together with the nursing process (which is most emphatically *not* a nursing model), they provide detailed guidance for the steps that need to be gone through when planning and delivering care.

Models of nursing, or 'conceptual models of nursing' as some authors call them, are built up out of concepts. In what has become a classic definition, Riehl and Roy describe a nursing model as:

a systematically constructed, scientifically based, and logically related set of concepts which identify the essential components of nursing practice together with the theoretical basis of these concepts and values required for their use by the practitioner. (1980: 6)

Several features of this definition are worthy of note. First, nursing models are *systematically* constructed. They are not simply personal opinions on how nursing should take place. Instead, they have been developed logically, with care and effort, in an attempt to provide guidance for the planning and delivery of nursing care. Second, they have *scientific foundations*, evolving from the observations that nurses make, from efforts to bring together ideas from existing fields of enquiry, or from both of these processes (Fawcett, 1995). Third, nursing models act as guides for *nursing practice* by suggesting better ways of nursing and caring for people. Fourth, they identify the values with which nurses should work, which is crucial if groups of nurses are to provide continuity of care. For example, nurses working with a model that values independence for patients should be encouraging this in their day-to-day practice.

Just like their physical counterparts, conceptual models have a number of components. We can call these the key components of care:

- The nature of people
- The causes of the problems likely to require nursing intervention
- The nature of assessment and nursing diagnosis
- The nature of planning and goal-setting
- The focus of intervention during the implementation of the care plan
- The nature of evaluation
- The role of the nurse.

The nature of people

Different nursing models make different assumptions about people and their health-related needs. Some see people in a way similar to the medical model – as interrelated sets of anatomical parts and physiological systems. Others suggest that it is not very helpful to 'fragment' people in this way, preferring to see individuals more holistically as 'whole beings' that are more than the sum of their parts. Other models of nursing emphasise the behavioural aspects of human beings, seeing them as people who can engage in different kinds of behaviour, some of which may be associated with particular health difficulties, others of which can lead to the restoration of well-being. Still other nursing models focus on the human ability to philosophise and give meaning to events and situations. Finally, there are models of nursing that work with ideas drawn from several of the above perspectives.

It is important to appreciate that models of nursing have their starting point in commonalities between people. Thus, the key component of *the nature of people* indicates those things which most people have in common. This should alert nurses to the danger of going too far towards the notion of individualised care. While people differ from one another, they are also very similar. Indeed, it is this similarity that allows nurses to learn from clinical experience and use this learning to inform future care.

The causes of problems likely to require nursing intervention

Just as nursing models differ in terms of the assumptions they make about the nature of people, so they vary in terms of what they see as being the most probable causes of the health-related problems that require nursing intervention. Some emphasise anatomical and physiological malfunctions, others focus more on the problems that arise when people fail to adopt behaviour appropriate to the circumstances in which they find themselves. Some highlight the difficulties that can arise when people come to perceive themselves and their health in ways that lead to maladaptation or imbalance, whereas others suggest that problems requiring nursing intervention are most likely to arise when the overall equilibrium between people and their environments becomes disturbed. Each model characterises the cause of health-related problems slightly differently, with consequent implications for the planning and delivery of care.

The nature of assessment and nursing diagnosis

Given the different ways in which models of nursing conceptualise people and the causes of health problems, it is not surprising that each emphasises different factors that should be attended to during nursing assessment and diagnosis. Models also differ in terms of their overall approach to assessment: some see it as a series of steps moving from a preliminary identification of problems to a more definite nursing diagnosis, others as a holistic, one-stage process.

The nature of planning and goal-setting

Another way in which nursing models differ is in terms of the planning that they advocate for nurses. While perhaps the majority of models are person centred in that they emphasise that the individual receiving care should be centrally involved in the planning of care, they differ in terms of their focus. Some argue that targets should be set for the return of function to parts of the body or physiological systems. Others argue that planning should focus on the restoration of equilibrium within a particular aspect of the patient's behaviour. Many advocate that nurses should pay particular attention to the setting of goals that relate to an individual's psychological or social well-being. Models differ, too, in terms of whether they advocate the setting of staged (short-term, intermediate and long-term) goals or whether they do not draw such distinctions. All models of nursing agree, however, that agreed goals should relate to observable aspects of the person's behaviour. When a goal has been achieved it should, therefore, be apparent from what that person says or does.

The focus of intervention during implementation of the care plan

By carrying out a systematic assessment and by setting realistic person-centred goals, the nurse will have begun to devise a plan of care. This will specify the aspects of the person that should be focused on in the delivery of nursing care, be these physiological or behavioural imbalances, inaccurate beliefs and perceptions, or deficits in self-care. Depending on the model being employed, different types of intervention will be appropriate in order to achieve the goals set in the care plan. Some models of nursing, for example, advocate holistic intervention aiming, perhaps, to restore an overall equilibrium between individuals and their environment. Others argue that particular physiological or behavioural systems should be targeted in nursing intervention. Still other models promote the use of nursing actions that help to alter how people see themselves and their health-related concerns.

What models of nursing do not do is to specify the particular actions that nurses should take to achieve agreed outcomes. Instead, they recommend types of activity in which nurses might engage. Nurses working with a specific model of nursing must select interventions from up-to-date, evidence-based practices, and should ultimately evaluate the effectiveness of their actions through summative evaluation and clinical supervision.

The nature of evaluation

Most nursing models emphasise the need to ensure that the outcomes of particular nursing interventions are compared against the goals originally set. When such goals appear not to have been met, the nurse should ask why this is so. Only by evaluating the extent to which goals have been achieved, and the appropriateness (or otherwise) of the interventions used, can we decide whether the approach to care employed has been appropriate. Formative evaluation of this kind is central to the application of all nursing models, but models differ in terms of the changes in behaviour that should be looked for. As before, some place importance on changes in bodily function whereas others recommend that particular attention be given to changes in psychological status, or to the extent to which an individual has been enabled to undertake self-care as a result of nursing intervention.

Formative evaluation of this kind is very different from summative evaluation. This takes place towards the close of a period of nursing intervention using a particular nursing model. It involves examining the extent to which the chosen model of nursing was appropriate for meeting the person's health-related needs. It may lead to the nurse concluding that an appropriate framework for the planning and delivery of care had been chosen, or it may encourage the use of an alternative model on a future occasion. Summative evaluation ideally should involve a number of nurses working together who have experience of using a particular model in a variety of circumstances.

The role of the nurse

Models of nursing differ from one another in terms of what they see as being the role of the nurse in the provision of care. In addition to acting as an assessor of needs, a planner, an intervener and an evaluator (roles suggested by the nursing process), the nurse is likely to have to adopt a more specialised overall role depending on the nature of the model of nursing being used. Examples of these overall roles include being a 'patient's advocate', a 'facilitator of self-care' or a 'modifier of behavioural patterns'. Nursing models are rarely neutral in what they have to say about the role of the nurse. The amount of shared decision-making advocated by a model, or alternatively its emphasis on the nurse taking control, tells us a great deal about the general commitments of any particular model of nursing.

Nursing theory

There has been much debate over what constitutes nursing theory. A variety of definitions abound, including the idea that it is a logically interconnected set of confirmed hypotheses (McKay, 1969), a conceptual framework invented for some purpose (Dickoff and James, 1968) and an imaginative grouping of knowledge, ideas and experience that are represented symbolically and seek to illuminate a given phenomenon (Watson, 1985). Following an extended examination of these and other definitions, Chinn and Kramer (1995: 72) conclude that a theory is 'a creative and rigorous structuring of ideas that project a tentative, purposeful and systematic view of phenomena'.

Some writers have distinguished between what are called different *levels of theory*: grand theory, which covers a wide range of issues; mid-range theory, which relates more to the needs and demands of nursing practice; micro-level theory, which relates only to very specific events and circumstances; and metatheory, this being theory about the process of theory development. Certainly, theories vary in their scope (the range of things that they explain) and their application (the range of circumstances in which they are useful), and there are important differences between theories that are highly specific and those which are more general.

But what is the relationship between theory and conceptual models of nursing? This is a question that has occupied the attention of many nurse writers and to which there is no clear-cut answer. On the one hand, there are those such as Meleis (1991: 16) who say that the 'differences are tentative at best and hair-splitting, unclear and confusing at worst'. On the other hand, there are others, for example Fawcett (1995), who believe that there are important differences between nursing models and nursing theories:

A conceptual model is an abstract and general system of concepts and propositions. A theory, in contrast, deals with one or more relatively specific and concrete concepts and propositions. Conceptual models are general guides that must be specified further by relevant and logically congruent theories before action can occur. (Fawcett, 1995: 27)

Conceptual models are therefore more abstract than theories. Because of this, they are rarely directly testable. Theories, on the other hand, describe, explain or predict relatively specific phenomena and events, and are thus more easily tested for their validity or their appropriateness. Conceptual models may act as the starting point for the development of nursing theory – they are not theories themselves, although they may contain the seeds of future ones.

Having clarified some of the differences between the nursing process, nursing models and nursing theory, we will now look in detail at a number of conceptual models of nursing. In doing this, the framework identified earlier will be used. In each case, we will begin by considering what that particular model has to say about people and their health care needs. We will begin our examination of different conceptual models by looking at an approach to care that, while likely to be familiar, does not derive from the insights of nurses or nurse theorists. This is the medical model of care. We begin here because of the influence that this approach has had, both on the work of doctors and on nursing itself.

After this, we will examine two models of nursing that borrow extensively from the medical model in terms of how they understand people and their health-related needs – the models of nursing suggested by Virginia Henderson and by Nancy Roper, Alison Tierney and Winfred Logan.

Following this, we will look at six models of nursing that pay greater attention to psychological and social needs while not ignoring the biological bases of behaviour – the nursing models developed by Dorothy Johnson, Callista Roy, Dorothea Orem, Imogene King, Hildegard Peplau and Betty Neuman.

We will then consider two models of nursing that depart more radically from dominant ways of seeing patients and nursing care. Joan Riehl-Sisca's model of nursing emphasises the human ability to 'philosophise' and make sense of situations, whereas Martha Rogers' holistic model of nursing offers an intellectually challenging way of understanding the relationship between people and their environments.

References

Bonney, V. and Rothenberg, J. (1963) *Nursing Diagnosis and Therapy: An Instrument for Evaluation and Measurement*. New York, The National League for Nursing.

Campbell, C. (1980) *Nursing Diagnosis and Intervention in Nursing Practice*. New York, Wiley.

Chinn P.L. and Kramer M.K. (1995) *Theory and Nursing: A Systematic Approach*, 4th edn. St Louis, C.V. Mosby.

Christenson, P. and Kenney, J. (1990) *Nursing Process: Application of Conceptual Models*. St Louis, C. V. Mosby.

Christenson, P. and Kenney, J. (1995) *Nursing Process: Application of Conceptual Models*, 4th edn. St Louis, C.V. Mosby.

Crow, J. (1977) The nursing process. *Nursing Times*, 73: 892–6.

Dickoff, J. and James, P. (1968) A theory of theories. *Nursing Research*, 17: 197–203.

Fawcett, J. (1995) *Analysis and Evaluation of Conceptual Models of Nursing*. Philadelphia, F.A. Davis.

George, J. (1995) *Nursing Theories: The Base for Professional Nursing Practice*. Norwalk, CT, Appleton & Lange.

Kelly, K. (1996) Clinical inference in nursing. *Nursing Research*, 15: 23.

Kratz, C. (1970) *The Nursing Process*. London, Baillière Tindall.

Linberg, J. Hunter, M. and Kruszewski, A. (1994) *Introduction to Nursing: Concepts, Issues and Opportunities*. Philadelphia, J.B. Lippincott.

Little, D. and Carnevali, D. (1971) *Nursing Care Planning*. Philadelphia, J.B. Lippincott.

Marriner, A. (1979) *The Nursing Process*. St Louis, C.V. Mosby.

Mayers, M. (1972) *A Systematic Approach to the Nursing Care Plan*. New York, Appleton-Century-Crofts.

McKay, R. (1969) *The Process of Theory Development in Nursing*. New York, Teachers College, Columbia University.

Meleis, A. (1991) *Theoretical Nursing: Development and Progress*. Philadelphia, J.B. Lippincott.

Oermann, M. (1991) *Professional Nursing Practice: A Conceptual Approach*. Philadelphia, J.B. Lippincott.

Riehl, J. and Roy, C. (eds) (1980) *Conceptual Models for Nursing Practice*, 2nd edn. Norwalk, CT, Appleton-Century-Crofts.

Watson, J. (1985) *Nursing – Human Science and Human Care: A Theory of Nursing*. Norwalk, CT, Appleton-Century-Crofts.

Wilkinson, J. (1992) *Nursing Process in Action: A Critical Thinking Approach*. Menlo Park, CA, Addison Wesley.

Yura, H. and Walsh, M. (1967) *The Nursing Process*. Norwalk, CT, Appleton-Century-Crofts.

Chapter 3 The medical model of care

In the previous chapter, we suggested some of the key concepts to be used throughout this book. We also described the key components likely to be found in any nursing model of care. Finally, we suggested that some nurses have welcomed the introduction of nursing models because they offer an understanding of people and their health-related needs that is distinct from that offered by the medical, natural and social sciences. Before examining a number of nursing models in detail, we will give a brief account of the medical model of care, an approach to health care delivery that will be familiar to most nurses. For many years, this has formed the basis of not only medical, but also nurse, training.

As a result of enquiry by social historians interested in medicine, it is now known that what counts as medicine varies dramatically over time and from place to place. What we understand by medicine today is, of course, a relatively recent set of health care practices, governed by a set of beliefs about people, health, illness and disease that would have appeared very strange a few hundred years ago.

Traditional ideas about health, illness and disease can be grouped into three relatively distinct perspectives: those offered by Chinese medicine, those offered by ayurvedic medicine, and those offered by European medicine up until the end of the eighteenth century (Aggleton, 1990). Each approach emphasises the fundamental wholeness of human beings – their *holism* – and the importance of *balance*, both within the person and between the person and his or her environment. Ayurvedic medicine, for example, lays emphasis on there being a balance between three bodily humours – wind (vayu), gall (pitta) and mucus (kapha) – whereas traditional European medicine has identified four such humours – blood, phlegm, yellow bile and black bile. The excess of any one of these humours is said to lead to sickness, the form of the illness being determined by the humour that is out of balance.

More recent medical explanations differ from these traditional ideas by distinguishing between the mind and the body, and between (1) *anatomical* parts (the heart, the brain, the liver, and so on), (2) *physiological* systems (the nervous system, the circulatory system, the respiratory system, and so on) and (3) the *biochemical* processes within these systems that may contribute to wellness or ill-health. Modern biomedicine, as it is sometimes called, emphasises the biological bases of behaviour. This can be seen in the emphasis given to the study of anatomy and physiology in initial medical training today, and by the fact that, among practising doctors, the causes of ill-health often come to be identified in terms of imbalances or defects within one or more of the above three aspects of human functioning.

When such ideas were first introduced in the sixteenth and seventeenth centuries, they aroused much controversy, not least because by suggesting that the causes of ill-health were pathogenic, dietary, environmental and emotional, they conflicted sharply with Christian teaching emphasising the links between sinful behaviour and being ill. Indeed, Vesalius' first anatomy textbook was denounced by the church in 1543, and strenuous efforts were made to prevent the dissection of the human body. This shows the power of vested interest in preserving the integrity of particular ways of thinking about health issues. It should thus come as little surprise to learn that the introduction of nursing models in the twentieth century has been seen by some as implying a questioning of modern medical authority.

Key components of care

The nature of people

According to the medical model, a person is a complex set of anatomical parts and physiological systems. While the functioning of these parts and systems may not be fully understood, it is believed that, in time, further biomedical research and scientific progress will lead to a better understanding of how they work. Within the medical model, much of a person's social behaviour and many psychological processes are thought to have their origins in physiological and biochemical activity. Mental illnesses such as depression may thus be related to imbalances between particular chemical transmitters in the brain, and drugs are prescribed to remedy the situation. Such a view, in which complex social behaviours are explained in terms of relatively simply biological processes, has been considered to be inadequate by many nurses and some doctors, who feel that it oversimplifies the nature of human behaviour and encourages a view of people as the 'passive hosts of disease' (Reynolds, 1985).

The causes of problems likely to require intervention

The medical model emphasises the existence of biological needs within people. Its emphasis on anatomical, physiological and biochemical malfunction as the causes of ill-health encourages a *disease-orientated* approach to care that stresses the structure and function of the body (and malfunctions within this) rather than the uniqueness or integrity of the individual (Thibodeau, 1983). Both physical and psychological health care problems are seen as arising when there is a malfunction within either an anatomical part or a physiological or biochemical system, or simultaneously in more than one of these.

The nature of assessment

Assessment using the medical model aims to identify what is *medically* wrong with the person. It focuses, therefore, on signs and symptoms. These are usually elicited by taking a medical history and by physically examining the person (most usually called the patient) in an attempt to identify those physiological or biochemical systems, or anatomical parts, in which there resides a malfunction. Ultimately, the process of assessment leads to a diagnosis being made. This diagnosis usually takes the form of a medical 'condition' and is usually named as such.

The nature of planning and goal-setting

Once the assessment has been completed, doctors and nurses working with the medical model of care plan to bring about change in particular bodily systems or parts. Frequently set goals include the restoration of previous levels of balance within particular systems and the return of function within particular parts. In contrast to many nursing models, goal-setting is rarely person centred. Instead it involves others (usually doctors) deciding what is the best strategy by which a malfunction within a system or part may be remedied and the associated medical condition cured.

The focus of intervention during implementation of the care plan

According to Burton (1985), intervention using the medical model mostly centres on 'putting things right'. Thus, it focuses not on the whole person, but on the physiological system or anatomical part that is perceived to have malfunctioned. It often involves prescribing or administering medication, or removing or modifying some anatomical part. The choice of intervention for a particular patient will depend both on the doctor's past experience of similar 'cases' and on the differences and needs of the individual, the former, however, being stressed by the medical model. Some interventions, or treatments, are so well established that doctors vary little in what they recommend (particular kinds of drug therapy or surgical procedure, for example). Others may be less so, and a considerable variation in treatment may be found. It is often difficult for the patient to know, however, whether or not a particular treatment is well established.

The nature of evaluation

Using the medical model, formative evaluation takes place by examining the extent to which prescribed interventions have been successful in meeting goals set for each physiological system or anatomical part deemed to have a malfunction. Summative evaluation, or reflection on the overall appropriateness of this broad approach to care, is less common. Ideally, however, it should involve a consideration of the extent to which this model, as opposed to others, has been appropriate in meeting a particular set of health care needs.

The role of the nurse

Nurses working with the medical model may find themselves little more than physicians' assistants, a role that has a long, if contested, tradition within nursing. As Chinn and Kramer (1995: 34) put it, traditionally 'nurses were expected to follow orders and serve the needs and interests of physicians providing care'. Doctors made the diagnoses and decided upon the action to be taken, nurses assisted in the delivery of care.

The past 20 years have seen modern biomedicine coming under increasing scrutiny, both in terms of its appropriateness as a system of beliefs to understand all health-related needs, and in terms of its capacity to fulfil increasing public expectations about health care provision. It is within this context that efforts by nurses to improve standards of care, including the introduction of nursing models and the nursing process, are perhaps best understood.

For writers such as Hall (1983: 466), efforts by nurses to improve health care services should not be 'seeking to erode the proper role of medical practitioners', but should instead complement the interventions that doctors make. Such a view presupposes, however, that there exists no inherent conflict between the purposes and practices of biomedicine and those advocated by particular models of nursing. As we will see, this may be a questionable assumption to make in relation to some models of nursing.

References

Aggleton, P.J. (1990) *Health*. London, Routledge.

Burton, M. (1985) The environment, good interaction and interpersonal skills in nursing. In Kagan, G. (ed.) *Interpersonal Skills in Nursing*. London, Croom Helm.

Chinn, P.L. and Kramer, M.K. (1995) *Theory and Nursing: A Systematic Approach*. St Louis, C.V. Mosby.

Hall, C. (1983) A time for reflection. *Journal of Advanced Nursing*, 8: 457–66.

Reynolds, B. (1985) Issues arising from teaching interpersonal skills in psychiatric nurse training. In Kagan, G. (ed.) *Interpersonal Skills in Nursing*. London, Croom Helm.

Thibodeau, J.A. (1983) *Nursing Models: Analysis and Evaluation*. Monterey, CA, Wadsworth Health Sciences Division.

Chapter 4 Henderson's model of nursing

Virginia Henderson qualified as a nurse in 1921 at the Army School of Nursing in Washington. Throughout much of her career, she worked as a nurse teacher and researcher, first at the Teachers' College at Columbia University and later at the prestigious Yale University. Her definition of nursing first appeared in print in 1955. Her pamphlet entitled *Basic Principles of Nursing Care* was published in 1960 by the International Council of Nurses (Henderson, 1960) and her book *The Nature of Nursing*, which describes the nurse's primary and unique function was published 6 years later (Henderson, 1966).

Henderson's own intellectual development was much influenced by contemporary developments in physiology and psychology. Through her physiology classes at the Teachers' College, Columbia University, Henderson learned of the importance of maintaining physiological balance or *homeostasis*, and through her work in psychology, she came to recognise people's fundamental psychological and social needs. Henderson believed that nurses need to pay particular care to accurately interpreting both verbal and non-verbal information from patients to avoid misconceiving and misinterpreting such needs. Her desire to individualise nursing care was informed by a discontent with the 'regimentalized patient care' in which she had earlier participated and 'the concept of nursing as merely ancillary to medicine' (Henderson 1966: 7). Virginia Henderson died in March 1996 at the age of 98.

Key components of care

The nature of people

According to Henderson, people have biological, psychological, social and spiritual components. Associated with each of these components are 14 fundamental human needs (Figure 4.1). The first nine of these are physiological; the tenth and fourteenth needs relate to the psychological functions of communicating and learning; the eleventh need is concerned with spirituality, and the twelfth and thirteenth needs with social aspects of life such as work and recreation. In health and sickness, people strive to satisfy these needs in various ways through 'infinitely varied patterns of living, no two of which are alike' (Henderson, 1960: 3).

1. To breathe normally
2. To eat and drink adequately
3. To eliminate body waste
4. To move and maintain desirable postures
5. To sleep and rest
6. To select suitable clothes – dress and undress
7. To maintain body temperature within the normal range
8. To keep the body clean and well groomed
9. To avoid changes in the environment and avoid injuring others
10. To communicate with others in expressing emotions, needs, fears and opinions
11. To worship according to one's faith
12. To work in such a way that there is a sense of accomplishment
13. To play or participate in various forms of recreation
14. To learn, discover or satisfy the curiosity that leads to normal development and health, and use available health facilities

Figure 4.1   Fundamental needs shared by all people

When people are well, they are unlikely to have much diffi-culty satisfying each of these needs themselves. However, in times of sickness, or at points in the life cycle such as childhood, preg-nancy or old age, or when death is approaching, an individual may be unable to satisfy these requirements without assistance from others. It is on such occasions that the nurse has a unique role to play in assisting the person to perform those activities which contribute to the recovery of health or a peaceful death.

At all times, nursing care aims to help people to regain inde-pendence as speedily as possible. The activities that nurses undertake relating to each need are described by Henderson as components of nursing. Fourteen sets of such nursing activities (or components of nursing) can be identified, one related to each basic need.

The causes of problems likely to require intervention

According to Henderson, nursing care is most usually needed when a person is unable to carry out activities contributing to health, recovery or a peaceful death. Special difficulties may arise, however, at particular stages in the life cycle. Those who are very young or very old, for example, may be unable to satisfy one or more of their basic needs because of physiological, psychological or social factors associated with their stage of development.

Physical and intellectual abilities can affect an individual's capacity to carry out activities to satisfy fundamental needs. People who are physically disabled, for example, through perhaps losing a special sense or a motor capacity, may require nursing care and assistance in order to satisfy fundamental needs such as moving and maintaining a desirable posture, as well as playing and participating in recreation. Some people with serious learning difficulties may benefit from nursing care in order to learn, discover and satisfy their curiosity.

Temperament and emotional state may also affect individuals' abilities to satisfy their fundamental needs. A highly anxious or frightened patient, for example, may experience problems with eating, drinking, sleeping and perhaps communicating. Many strong emotional reactions are triggered by social and environmental cues linked to the circumstances in which people find themselves. Nurses thus have an important role to play in organising the environment around patients in order to minimise the likelihood of negative temperamental and emotional reactions.

Further problems can arise from the social and cultural status of the individual. An elderly person, recently bereaved and living alone, may have difficulty moving around the house, selecting suitable clothing and communicating in the absence of the help and support previously provided by a relative or friend. A younger person who is homeless and perhaps living rough on the streets may have difficulty eating and drinking adequately, keeping her body clean and well groomed, and perhaps communicating with others in expressing her needs, fears and opinions.

Physical, psychological and social factors such as those discussed limit the individual's ability to carry out activities that lead to the recovery of health. Nursing care is needed to make whole or complete those needs which are unfulfilled.

The nature of assessment

Henderson advocates a deliberative approach to assessment. This involves the nurse assessing the patient in relation to each of the 14 components of basic nursing care. Assessment should involve communication and negotiation since only in highly dependent states such as coma or extreme prostration would the nurse be justified in deciding for, rather than with, the patient what is good for him.

An empathetic approach to assessment is advocated in which the nurse tries to see things from the patient's point of view. While Henderson does not explicitly argue for it, her model suggests the value of a two-stage assessment. In the first stage, the nurse might work with the patient, considering in turn each fundamental need that might or might not be satisfied at present. Together, nurse and patient must decide, for each of these needs, whether nursing assistance is needed.

In a second stage, they must decide what is causing the problems that demand nursing care. This involves deciding for each unmet fundamental need whether the causes are primarily physiological, psychological, social or spiritual in nature. Only on this basis can effective interventions be planned.

The nature of planning and goal-setting

For Henderson, planning and goal-setting should be patient centred, involving efforts by the nurse to 'get inside [the patient's] skin' (Henderson, 1966: 24). In many nursing contexts, it may be appropriate to set short-term, intermediate and long-term goals. The latter most usually involve helping the patient to regain complete independence where possible with respect to fundamental human needs. Short-term and intermediate goals, on the other hand, generally relate to the causes of problems identified during assessment and are likely to take account of pathological states or syndromes such as infection, fever, dehydration and shock.

Since Henderson believes that nursing care is something to be carried out in conjunction with the treatments provided by medically qualified personnel, the plan of nursing care should explicitly include drugs and treatments prescribed by the physician. In this respect, Henderson's model of nursing differs from some others in that it explicitly acknowledges the complementary relationship between nursing and medical care.

The focus of intervention during implementation of the care plan

Once short-term, intermediate and long-term goals have been set, nursing intervention can take place. The majority of interventions made by nurses using Henderson's model aim to substitute for what the patient lacks in relation to one or more identified needs. Three different kinds of nurse–patient relationship can be identified, each with its own type of intervention (Alexander *et al.*, 1998). First, the nurse can act as a *substitute* for the patient; second, she can act as a *helper* for the patient; and third, she can act as a *partner*. Which of these styles of intervention is adopted depends on the nature of the nurse–patient relationship.

Using Henderson's model, interventions should be individualised in order to take into account the unique aspects of the patient's physiological, psychological and social well-being. The patient's desire to depend on others should be acknowledged when this is appropriate, for example in conditions of serious illness.

The nature of evaluation

Within this model of nursing, evaluation involves examining the extent to which, following intervention, a patient has been helped by the nurse to meet fundamental needs that were in some way unmet before nursing intervention took place. In the short term, evaluation should focus on the extent to which goals, agreed upon between patient and nurse, have been met. This kind of formative evaluation can help the nurse to revise the care plan drawn up with a particular individual. In the longer term, evaluation should look at the extent to which the patient can perform independently following nursing intervention.

Summative evaluation will need to be conducted over a more prolonged period of time and with a number of patients. It involves reaching decisions about the overall usefulness of Henderson's model of nursing within a particular nursing setting or in meeting a specific type of patient need.

The role of the nurse

Henderson describes in her writing several roles for the nurse that fit together perhaps rather uneasily. On the one hand, she is at pains to emphasise the unique function of the nurse as an independent health care professional. As she puts it:

The unique function of the nurse is to assist the individual sick or well, in the performance of those activities contributing to health and its recovery (or to peaceful death) that he would perform unaided if he had the necessary strength, will or knowledge. And to do this in such a way as to help him gain independence as rapidly as possible. (Henderson, 1966: 15)

This definition, which defines nursing in terms of *functions*, Henderson found useful in that it focused attention on what nurses do in order to assist people, be they sick or well, in gaining or regaining their independence.

On the other hand, and despite her personal distaste for regimented and non-individualised systems of care, Henderson identified a more stereotyped nursing role, that of the physician's helper, along with the allied possibility of nursing goals being subsumed within a medical plan of treatment. She describes it thus:

the nursing history parallels the medical history; the nurse's health assessment, the physician's medical examination; the nursing diagnosis corresponds to the physician's diagnosis; nursing orders to the plan of medical management; and nursing evaluation to medical evaluation (Henderson, 1980: 907).

Whether these two roles are so complementary as to be subsumed one within the other remains to be seen. There can be little doubt, however, that Henderson's model of nursing did much to lay the foundations for the development of subsequent conceptual frameworks for the planning and application of nursing care.

Using Henderson's model

Like most nursing models that originated in the 1960s, Henderson's model conceptualises the role and function of the nurse as a means of restoring people to health or maximising their sense of well-being. For Henderson, independence is largely seen as being synonymous with health and well-being. Despite the familiarity of this model to many nurses, some suggestions will be made about its use with the nursing process in planning and delivering care. Of the two examples chosen, one will focus on the restoration of health while the other will consider the needs of a healthy individual at an important stage of the life cycle. As has been identified above, people may not be able to satisfy their fundamental needs unaided in times of sickness or when significant life changes are occurring.

It should be borne in mind that Henderson's model of nursing works with a firm commitment to patient participation in care, and this is likely to have implications for all four stages of the nursing process.

Assessment – first stage

The first stage of the process of patient assessment is likely to identify those fundamental needs which are not being met. In most instances, nurse and patient should reach agreement about these, the nurse only deciding on behalf of patients when they are unable to participate in the process.

With increased longevity, more people are experiencing some loss of independence as a result of a variety of degenerative changes. Nurses may thus be involved in planning and delivering care to people with difficulties meeting their needs for movement and maintaining a desirable posture. An example might be that of an elderly woman admitted to hospital prior to elective surgery to replace a damaged hip joint. Together, the nurse and patient may identify that the fundamental need related to movement (Henderson's fourth fundamental need) is not being met, or that movement is only achieved with some discomfort. In addition, the nurse will want to consider the patient's views about how well other related needs are being met, for example the need to dress and undress (sixth fundamental need) and the needs for a sense of accomplishment and for recreation (twelfth and thirteenth fundamental needs respectively).

Nursing knowledge will also suggest that the nurse explores with the patient her knowledge of the planned surgical procedure so that preoperative information can be given to benefit the patient's recovery (Hayward, 1975; Boore, 1978; Gammon and Mulholland, 1996). Thus, the fourteenth fundamental need will also be important when beginning this assessment.

A community midwife might also find it useful to pay attention to the need for learning in order to assist normal development when helping young women and their partners to prepare for childbirth. For example, during a home visit to a woman of African descent who has not lived in this country long, discussion might take place about a number of fundamental needs. However, the woman might express particular concern about how prepared she feels for the changes taking place to her body and for her development into the role of a mother. Together, the midwife and pregnant woman might identify the importance of the fourteenth fundamental need to her immediate care.

Assessment – second stage

Once the areas of chief concern have been identified and the relevant fundamental needs highlighted, the nurse or midwife will proceed to the second stage of the assessment process with the patient. Here, the aim will be to decide the probable causes of the patient's unmet needs so that realistic goals can be set.

To return to the woman approaching surgery to replace her hip joint, she and the nurse are likely to focus on any particular movements or manoeuvres that cause discomfort so that these can, as far as possible, be avoided in the preoperative period. Degenerative changes cannot usually be altered by nursing care, but discomfort can often be alleviated. Therefore, nurses and surgeons each have a role in helping patients to be independent.

Henderson's model may seem especially apt here because, in her writing about nursing, Henderson acknowledges the role of the nurse *vis-à-vis* other health professionals, especially doctors. Her claim that nursing care should always be arranged around, or fitted into, the physician's therapeutic plan sits uneasily with many nurses' view of autonomous practice today. Patients undergoing surgical procedures require a collaborative approach to intervention on the part of both nurses and surgeons if care is to be consistent and of a high quality. The relationship can often be one of more mutual respect than is implied by Henderson's work.

The pregnant woman may be preparing for her first child without the support of other close family members. She may express concern that she is missing the learning opportunities normally provided in her culture by contact with other family relations, particularly women. She may also feel unsure about how childbirth and child care are managed in this country and have anxieties about preserving the important cultural heritage of her background.

Planning care

Henderson's commitment to the notion of an individual independently fulfilling fundamental human needs means that the long-term goal for nursing care will be for the person once more to gain independence with respect to these needs. To achieve this, and taking note of all the information gathered during assessment, nurses are likely to negotiate with the patient several short-term and intermediate goals.

Thus, the nurse working with the woman preparing for hip surgery may suggest that, in the short term, goals are related to the relief of pain when moving. However, she is also likely to consider the management of discomfort and pain, and the initial limitations on movement in the immediate postoperative period, and to discuss intermediate goals related to this. Setting postoperative goals at this time should also highlight the need to plan for a discussion of various aspects of the surgical treatment and aftercare. Planning can thus incorporate the important fourteenth fundamental need by looking forward to the goals of the early postoperative period and using their identification as a way of including the patient's need for information. Henderson recognised that the nurse would often be involved in teaching as an important part of the care plan (Henderson, 1969).

Similarly, the midwife may discuss with the woman expecting a baby ways in which she would be happy to learn more about childbirth and child care. First, they may together construct a list of short-term goals, which might include knowledge to be gained and skills to be acquired. Drawing on her own knowledge of learning theory, the midwife can offer alternative ways of achieving the agreed goals.

For example, the midwife might suggest attendance at antenatal classes or access to explanatory leaflets. The woman's cultural background will be particularly relevant here, and the midwife may be able to provide information about the types of activity that take place at antenatal classes. With this information, the woman may judge whether or not the classes seem sensitive to cultural difference. The midwife may know of written information that has proved helpful to African women from the same background, or may know a midwife or health visitor who has a similar cultural background and who could be involved in the planned interventions.

Intermediate goals may focus on the level of confidence expressed by the woman concerning her ability to function independently as she approaches the birth.

Patient-centred goals set while planning care should be realistic and should look forward to the evaluation stage of the nursing process by identifying those behaviours which may later be observed and/or measured to evaluate the success (or otherwise) of nursing intervention. The nurse caring for the woman with degenerative change in the hip joint might suggest the use of a pain chart as a means of monitoring some aspects of goal attainment. The midwife is likely to rely particularly on the woman's verbal expressions of confidence in assuming her new role and in her demonstration of any relevant practical skills.

Nursing intervention and the delivery of care

Henderson's model of nursing is not very explicit with respect to recommended nursing interventions, although other writers, including George (1995) and Adam (1980), have suggested a number of ways of intervening that may be appropriate for use with this model. These include positively reinforcing the patient, getting to know him better, completing tasks for him and increasing the supply of factors needed for recovery to health. In addition, as has been identified, Henderson accepts the idea that nursing should be organised around medical interventions, and this may also suggest some activities in which nurses might engage. For example, nurses working in surgical settings may help to prepare people for surgical interventions, and many nurses give medications prescribed by physicians. It is not always clear how such interventions link with the goals for care agreed by patient and nurse together, but it seems likely that Henderson would have approved of such activities.

More important is Henderson's view of the value of physical nursing care as part of the nursing role, and of the dangers of delegating this to unqualified carers:

They [unqualified nurses] may fail to assess the patient's needs adequately but, perhaps more important, the qualified nurse, being deprived of the opportunity while giving physical care to assess his needs, may not find any other chance to do so. (Henderson, 1960: 10–11)

An endorsement such as this of the value of care being given by qualified nurses is probably more important than ever today. Financial pressures within health care have made the use of unqualified, and therefore cheaper, carers seem especially attractive to managers. As has been argued elsewhere (Chalmers, 1995), qualified nurses have accountability for the delivery of nursing care, and it is difficult to exercise this when the nurse is not the direct care-giver.

For the woman preparing for surgery to her hip, the nurse may learn more about her coping strategies at home and may advocate the continuance of any pain-relieving drugs, or other interventions, already found to be effective. The nurse may also be able to complete any particularly uncomfortable tasks for the patient, perhaps tasks related to the sixth fundamental need of dressing and undressing, to minimise pain in the preoperative period spent in hospital.

Additionally, the nurse may supply factors designed to aid recovery to health and independence. For example, opportunities could be provided for the woman to practise certain skills related to movement (fourth fundamental need) that should benefit her in the first few days following surgery. She may practise rolling in bed with the aid of an Immoturn or try lifting herself using a 'monkey pole'.

The midwife's input may also help the woman to gain confidence and independence as she approaches childbirth and her new role as a mother. She may facilitate her joining an antenatal class or provide information through written material or through an introduction to a knowledgeable colleague. She will also be able to positively reinforce knowledge gained and skills acquired. Regular meetings could occur at which the woman talks with the midwife about the learning that has taken place. Positive reinforcement might well take the form of verbal praise.

Nursing interventions should seek to achieve realistic levels of independence. It is not to be expected that, prior to surgery or immediately afterwards, the woman will be completely independent with respect to movement (fourth fundamental need) or to her fundamental need to learn new things about the management of her health following a hip replacement (fourteenth fundamental need).

Henderson acknowledges that family members have a role to play in the delivery of care, although she remains relatively non-explicit about the manner in which they might contribute. It might be important for the midwife to include the woman's partner in the planned interventions. In this example, some aspects of the plan may involve the partner explicitly. He may attend classes as well, or he may be an important person to provide additional positive reinforcement for confidence gained.

Evaluation

In formatively evaluating the care given to patients, nurses are likely to use their care plans to determine how far the goals set at the planning stage have been met. Nurses working with Henderson's model of nursing, in particular, are likely to begin a formative evaluation of their care by re-examining each fundamental need diagnosed during assessment as being incompletely met by the person's own resources. The nurse will then look at the extent to which goals relating to each need have been satisfied. For every unmet goal, new nursing interventions may be identified, or the goal itself may be reformulated to allow a greater potential for success in subsequent nursing care.

Thus, the nurse caring for the woman with a painful hip may look particularly at the pain chart to evaluate the success of care aimed at alleviating pain associated with movement. She may also discuss with the woman whether she feels able to move independently and without pain sufficiently for her other needs, or whether certain activities remain problematic. In the short period of hospitalisation usually required before surgery, the patient may be happy to avoid some of her normal activities in order to be relatively pain-free.

The evaluation of some of the preoperative interventions will necessarily be delayed until the operation has taken place. In particular, the degree of independence of movement associated with the use of mobility aids will probably not be first evaluated until the second postoperative day.

Evidence of goal attainment for the pregnant woman is likely to take special note of her own feelings about her knowledge of the bodily changes that take place during and after pregnancy and her confidence to assume the role of mother and child carer. At assessment, it was the woman herself who identified the unmet fourteenth fundamental need, and it will be her views that should be paramount in evaluating the success of the midwife's interventions. Later evaluation may consider her feelings after the baby is born and how well she feels she copes during the first few weeks. The midwife is likely to be particularly keen to know how well the planned interventions demonstrated sensitivity to, and an understanding of, the woman's cultural background.

Summative evaluation of Henderson's model of nursing can only take place after it has been worked with for some time in a particular nursing or midwifery context. In carrying out this type of evaluation, nurses and midwives are likely to explore the effectiveness of this particular model of care, compared with others, in meeting the needs of a wide range of patients in that setting. In addition, thought should be given to how relevant the concept of independence seems to be for the patient group. Practitioners may also want to enquire whether working with this particular nursing model gives them sufficient autonomy as members of the health-care team.

References

Adam, E. (1980) *To be a Nurse*. Eastbourne, W.B. Saunders.

Alexander, J.E., Wertman DeMeester, D., Lauer, T. *et al*. (1998) Virginia Henderson. Definition of nursing. In Tomey, A.M. and Alligood, M.R. (eds) *Nursing Theorists and Their Work*, 4th edn. St Louis, C.V. Mosby.

Boore, J. (1978) *Prescription for Recovery*. RCN Research Series. London, RCN.

Chalmers, H. (1995) *Accountability in Nursing Models and the Nursing Process*. In Watson, R. (ed.) *Accountability in Nursing Practice*. London, Chapman & Hall.

Gammon, J. and Mulholland, C.W. (1996) Effect of preparatory information prior to elective total hip replacement on psychological coping outcomes. *Journal of Advanced Nursing*, 24: 303–8.

George, J. (1995) *Nursing Theories: The Base for Professional Nursing Practice*. London, Prentice Hall International.

Hayward, J. (1975) *Information: A Prescription Against Pain*. RCN Nursing Care Series. London, RCN.

Henderson, V. (1960) *Basic Principles of Nursing Care*. Geneva, International Council of Nurses.

Henderson, V. (1966) *The Nature of Nursing: A Definition and its Implications for Practice, Research and Education*. New York, Macmillan.

Henderson, V. (1969) *Basic Principles of Nursing Care*. Geneva, International Council of Nurses.

Henderson, V. (1980) Nursing – yesterday and tomorrow. *Nursing Times*, 76: 905–7.

Chapter 5 Roper, Logan and Tierney's activities of living model of nursing

Nancy Roper trained as a nurse at the Leeds General Infirmary and later worked as Principal Tutor at the Cumberland Infirmary School of Nursing, and at the Scottish Home and Health Department. Winifred Logan also undertook her initial training as a nurse at the Leeds General Infirmary. She later taught nursing at the University of Edinburgh and worked at the Scottish Home and Health Department, where she was responsible for nursing education. She then became Head of the Department of Nursing and Health Studies at Glasgow College of Technology. Alison Tierney graduated from the BSc in Social Science and Nursing course and undertook postgraduate study at the University of Edinburgh. After teaching nursing at this same university, she was appointed director of the university's Nursing Research Unit.

The foundations for what was later to become the Roper, Logan and Tierney (R–L–T) model of nursing were laid in the late 1970s in a study of the clinical experience of learner nurses conducted by Nancy Roper (1976). She was particularly interested in developing an image or idea about nursing that would help learners to look beyond the medical labels attached to patients in order to see the living person as a whole. For Roper, daily living activities were an important way of identifying the common nursing requirements shared by all patients. The basic framework for the R–L–T model of nursing was spelled out in several books published in the 1980s, including *The Elements of Nursing* (Roper *et al.*, 1980), *Learning to Use the Process of Nursing* (Roper *et al.*, 1981) and *Using a Model of Nursing* (Roper *et al.*, 1983). Throughout these publications, and in third (or fourth) editions of some of them, the model has been subsequently refined and developed. Specific modifications include a progressive move away from a disease-based approach to care, a redefinition of nursing to emphasise its role in preventing, alleviating or coping with problems of activities of living, and a greater awareness of the cultural, environmental, political and economic factors affecting health.

Key components of care

The nature of people

The starting point for the R–L–T model of nursing lies in the well-known hierarchy of human needs identified by the psychologist Abraham Maslow (1954). This orders human needs from the most basic to the most sophisticated. In this theory, unless basic physiological and safety needs such as the need for food, water, air and shelter are met, people cannot go on to express themselves in intellectual, artistic and creative endeavours. Only when this happens are the foundations for 'self-actualisation' present.

This hierarchy of needs to some extent underpins Henderson's notion of 14 universal human needs described in the previous chapter. In contrast to Henderson, however, Roper was keen to emphasise the *active* qualities of human beings and their interactions with one another and with the environment (Newton, 1991). Hence, in the R–L–T model, people are best understood in terms of the activities they carry out. Roper (1976) herself originally identified 16 activities of daily living (ADLs). Some of these are essential to the maintenance of human life, whereas others enhance the quality of life but are not essential for it. One (dying) is given special attention since it is the final act of living in which a person engages (Figure 5.1).

This early list of behaviours was later refined to specify 12 activities of living (ALs), these being central to the model in its later versions. Each AL specifies a relatively distinct type of human behaviour related to meeting a particular need (Figure 5.2). Some ALs have a biological basis. Those linked to eating, drinking and breathing are like this. Others are more socially and culturally determined: ALs relating to personal dress, cleanliness, work/play and sexuality are more of this kind.

People differ in the ways in which they involve themselves in ALs. Very young people and very old people, for example, may have difficulty performing particular ALs. Roper *et al.* therefore identify an independence–dependence continuum in their model, an individual's placement on this continuum depending, for example, on maturity, social and economic circumstances, and cultural background. It is important to recognise, however, that while some people may not involve themselves in certain ALs through personal choice, others may be unable to do so through lack of social or economic opportunity.

Essential	Breathing
	Eating
	Eliminating
	Controlling body temperature
	Mobilising
	Sleeping
	Fulfilling safety and security needs
Increased quality of living	Personal cleansing
	Dressing
	Communicating
	Learning
	Working
	Playing
	Sexualising
	Procreating
Mortality	Dying

Figure 5.1   Activities of daily living

1. Maintaining a safe environment
2. Communicating
3. Breathing
4. Eating and drinking
5. Eliminating
6. Personal cleansing and dressing
7. Controlling body temperature
8. Mobilising
9. Working and playing
10. Expressing sexuality
11. Sleeping
12. Dying

Figure 5.2   Activities of living

Three further types of activity are described in the R–L–T model: preventing, comforting and seeking behaviours. These are all related to the maintenance or restoration of health and include actions that reduce health risks, behaviours that make oneself or others feel better, and activities that may help to gain access to information of future health benefit. While not extensively referred to in writing about the model, these behaviours are important in that they specify a range of behaviours in which both nurses and patients may participate throughout a period of care.

The causes of problems likely to require intervention

A wide range of factors can give rise to problems that call for nursing intervention. These include the developmental stage that the person has reached and also encompass life events (such as pregnancy or infertility) linked to one of these stages. Eight developmental stages are described in the model: prenatal, infancy (birth to 5 years), childhood (6–12 years), adolescence (13–18 years), early adulthood (19–30 years), middle years (31–45 years), late adulthood (46–65 years) and old age (66 and above). They match closely those described by the psychologist Erickson (1950). Physical, psychological, sociocultural, environmental and politico-economic factors may also result in a need for nursing intervention. Among the physical factors identified by the R–L–T model as influencing nursing need are disability and disturbed physiology, pathological and degenerative tissue change, and accident and infection. Among the relevant psychological factors are intelligence, motivation and emotional state. Socio-cultural factors include religious beliefs and cultural norms such as those influencing eating and drinking. Environmental and political factors include the accessibility to and distribution of key resources for health. The absence of one or more of these factors may move the individual from relative independence to relative dependence for one or more AL.

The nature of assessment

The R–L–T model of nursing suggests that assessment should be an active process carried out around ALs. It is likely to involve the nurse and patient considering each activity in turn in order to identify previous routines and coping mechanisms as well as actual or potential nursing problems. Sometimes assessment will involve consideration of all the ALs specified by the model. On other occasions, the nurse may focus on certain ALs in accordance with the nursing actions available in a particular setting. Opinions differ on how inclusive assessment should aim to be. Roper *et al.* (1983) clearly state that it may not be necessary to consider each AL in a patient assessment, whereas Newton (1991) argues that, with the exception of 'dying', every AL should be taken into account. In circumstances in which no problems can be identified with a particular AL, the nurse should record a statement to this effect.

Other nursing problems that require identification during assessment are those which derive from the treatments prescribed by medical and other health professionals. These, too, should be identified since they may influence the plans that nurses make and the actions they take in delivering care. They constitute what the R–L–T model calls the medically prescriptive component of nursing.

The nature of planning and goal-setting

In order for the goals of nursing care to be realistic and achievable, they must be set in partnership with the patient. This involves good two-way communication. Without this, there is no guarantee that what the nurse believes could be achieved will match what the patient desires to attain. Goals should relate to how independent or dependent the patient is in relation to specified ALs, and should identify observable and measurable changes in this independence or dependence. Both long-term and short-term goals may be negotiated, although the model gives special emphasis to those which are of short duration. Goal-setting in relation to one AL may have consequences for planning in the next. Care should be taken, therefore, to ensure that complementary goals are set.

Subsequent to goal-setting, attention should be given to the personnel, equipment and resources that can be mobilised for patient care. Some consideration of alternative strategies may need to take place in order that informed choices can be made, and in order to avoid acting simply in accordance with past precedent in that particular nursing setting. A care plan should be drawn up that reflects negotiated goals for each relevant AL and the actions it is planned to take to meet these.

The focus of intervention during implementation of the care plan

A range of nursing actions may be used in order to help patients to meet the goals negotiated with them, although it should be recognised that the R–L–T model, like other models of nursing, provides only guidance on the appropriate actions to take. Relevant actions may include the preventive, comforting and seeking behaviours previously described. A nurse may act to prevent certain situations arising, for example, or she may comfort the patient physically and mentally. Alternatively, she may seek to minimise the patient's dependence so that she or he can seek greater responsibility for self-care. Wherever possible, nursing actions should be organised around current ALs and should seek to build upon these wherever possible, it often being easier to modify an existing behaviour than to substitute a new one.

Nursing interventions may also need to be made in relation to medically prescribed care, and this in turn may have consequences for the patient's ability to carry out particular ALs. This is one reason why care plans may need regular revision in order to make allowance for the anticipated and unanticipated nursing consequences of medically prescribed care. For example, patients may gain relief from certain oral pain-relieving drugs but may at the same time develop constipation.

The nature of evaluation

Patient behaviours or activities decided upon during planning and goal-setting are the criteria to be used in evaluating the care delivered. Many of these will relate to changes in independence or dependence for a particular AL and can be measured accordingly. Progress in meeting goals such as communicating, engaging in leisure pursuits (playing) and expressing oneself sexually can be assessed directly through observation, and indirectly through the accounts that patients give of their experiences. When expected outcomes do not take place, joint reassessment should occur. This may lead to problems being redefined and/or different goals being set.

Summative evaluation, on the other hand, involves a consideration of the extent to which the R–L–T model is valuable for use within a particular setting. It can only be undertaken once a number of nurses have worked with the model and when the results of several more formative evaluations are available. From within nursing, the view has been expressed that evaluation is relatively underemphasised in some presentations of the R–L–T model (Wilson-Barnett, 1981), and while the model enjoys good acceptability among nurses in Britain, it has not been subjected to sustained evaluation.

The role of the nurse

Roper *et al.* (1985) specify independent, dependent and interdependent roles for the nurse. A nurse may be independent when, as an independent practitioner, she comforts the patient. She is dependent when carrying out care prescribed by doctors or other health professionals, or when contributing to the alleviation or cure of medically defined conditions. She may be interdependent when she works together with other members of the health care team to meet goals requiring input of several different kinds, or when carrying out preventive actions as part of health education or health promotion.

Using Roper, Logan and Tierney's model

As stated earlier, Roper *et al.* place considerable emphasis on the ALs that people carry out. Indeed, they see a knowledge of these activities as a means of understanding people. This does not mean, however, that the model is only appropriate for those whose difficulties seem to be largely physical in nature. What it does mean is that nurses can use the knowledge gained about someone's ALs as a way of achieving a more in-depth understanding of that person's needs. To illustrate this, one example of using the R–L–T model in practice, in conjunction with the nursing process, will focus on bereavement. The other example will consider someone with more physical difficulties admitted for respite care.

Assessing

Roper *et al.* have long argued for the use of the word 'assessing' in preference to 'assessment', and this remains their position in the most recent edition of *The Elements of Nursing* (Roper *et al.*, 1996). For them, use of the word 'assessing' signifies the ongoing nature of the activity. By repeatedly assessing and reviewing patients and their needs, nurses are likely to gain a greater insight into the nature of problems affecting those in their care. With this model of nursing, assessing includes (Roper *et al.*, 1996: 52):

- collecting information from/about the person
- reviewing the collected information
- identifying the person's problems
- identifying priorities among problems.

Despite arguing for ongoing assessment, Roper *et al.* do suggest a two-stage process, initial assessment establishing baseline information against which further information can be compared; data about the person's usual routines and current problems in relation to the ALs can then be added to this.

The second stage of nursing assessment should focus on the individual's ability to carry out the 12 ALs. While Roper *et al.* have suggested that there are circumstances in which it might be appropriate to consider only a few of these activities in assessing patient needs, it is likely that some assessment of each will be necessary before a nurse can safely ignore any one of them. When possible, information should be gathered from and verified with the person being assessed, but there are occasions when secondary sources, such as people who know the patient well, may add to the available data.

Assessing – first stage

While acknowledging that assessment data should be gathered as soon as possible, Roper *et al.* (1996) recognise that, in some instances, it may be several hours before detailed information is available. They also recognise that, in emergency situations, priority will be given to the need for certain information, often of a physical nature. Ideally, however, they advocate collecting biographical and health data first. Such information includes personal details such as name, people important to the individual being assessed, religious beliefs and significant life crises.

For a woman whose husband has recently died in a hospice, a nurse may already have some of this information, gathered earlier as part of the care of the dying man and his family. To offer ongoing support, however, some information of importance will need to be verified and some new data may be forthcoming. For example, the husband's death will be a recent life crisis, and its significance to his wife may be crucial to how she copes during the early stages of bereavement and afterwards. The emotions that might be felt following the death of a loved one should not be assumed by the nurse but need to be ascertained during a careful and sensitive initial assessment:

sometimes death brings relief to those left behind and this may be the case, for example, if the family has had to watch suffering in someone they love, and bear the burden of care during a prolonged terminal illness. (Roper *et al.*, 1996: 398)

The importance of other relationships will also have a bearing on the support that might be needed from the hospice nurse. Earlier data may need to be checked as those most able to offer support during the husband's illness may not be the same people to whom the wife will now turn for help.

For an elderly man with transient lower limb weakness admitted for respite care, personal information will also need to include his usual living accommodation and any support services currently being utilised. Health records from the community nurse, for example, may be an invaluable secondary source of information. Today's emphasis on the need to begin discharge planning at an early stage in inpatient care is particularly important in respite care nursing, which provides an opportunity not only for family members to be temporarily relieved of the burden of care, but also for a detailed reassessment of a person's capabilities and problems. As such, respite care should be regarded as more than giving respite, although attention is also needed to ensure that assessment takes into account the patient's usual environment and does not exclusively focus on those activities which can or cannot be carried out independently in the inpatient setting.

Assessing – second stage

During the second stage of assessment, nurses will look particularly at the individual's ability to carry out the 12 ALs and to what degree they can each be carried out independently. Attention should always be paid to the person's usual routines and coping strategies so that nursing care can be individualised and as minimally disruptive to the person's normal mode of living as possible. The quality of the data gathered at assessment should ensure that goals set during the planning phase are realistic and attainable. The result of the second stage of assessing is the identification of actual and/or potential problems.

A hospice nurse assessing a woman following the death of her husband will need to consider the potential or actual impact of bereavement on the woman's ALs. In particular, information might be collected about dying (AL 12), expressing sexuality (AL 10) and sleeping (AL 11), although no activity should be ignored because bereavement and grief can have a profound effect on a person's ability to do many things for him or herself.

Thus, for example, the nurse and woman might discuss what impact her husband's death has had on the woman's feelings about death and dying. Such a discussion may focus both on the events that preceded the recent death and on how the woman now feels about her own mortality and about the lack of her partner as she grows older. Her position on the lifespan continuum may particularly influence thoughts about her own death, and an actual or potential problem may be identified related to fear of dying alone.

Assessing the AL related to expressing sexuality could involve the hospice nurse gaining an understanding of the particular activities the woman engaged in with her husband that she felt enabled her to express her sexuality. Adults who have lost a partner often notice especially the loss of physical touch with someone they love. There could be an actual problem of having less opportunity for loving, physical contact.

The woman might also express concern at her own changed sleep pattern or about vivid dreams depicting her husband as still being alive. The lack of sleep might be an actual problem, with the potential for distress from disturbing dreams.

The man with transient weakness of his legs may have problems in a number of ALs but particularly in mobilising (AL 8), maintaining a safe environment (AL 1) and working and playing

(AL 9). While at first glance these activities may look as though they are physical in nature and directly caused by the man's limb weakness, a careful second stage assessment is required to gain information about the nature of the influencing factors.

A feature of the R–L–T model that is crucial to understanding someone's abilities with regard to all the ALs is the influence of the five groups of named factors: biological, psychosocial, socio-cultural, environmental and politico-economic. In the example of the man with transient limb weakness, an actual problem with mobility (AL 8) could be the direct result of a loss of strength in his legs, and this would constitute a biological influencing factor. However, the inpatient setting might not provide an environment for walking that offers him sufficient, familiar help (enviromental and psychological influencing factors). At home, for example, there might be items of furniture or handrails positioned for his individual needs so that he can be independently mobile with confidence in some parts of the house.

Similarly, a nurse assessing his ability to maintain a safe environment (AL 1) will collect information of relevance both to the inpatient setting and to his home enviroment in preparation for his safe discharge. She will need to know whether he can summon assistance when required while in her care and also when at home. She may ask him to demonstrate his ability to use the call bell system and discuss those occasions on which he will need help from a nurse to remain safe. For example, he may always need help to get safely into bed. The nurse may record information about his methods of summoning assistance when at home and identify a potential problem when family members are not within hearing distance.

There are likely to be marked differences in the opportunities for activities related to working and playing (AL 9) in hospital and in a home setting. Roper *et al.* (1996) stress the importance of challenge and achievement for the satisfaction of this AL, and respite care might be used to reassess the man's ability to engage in chosen activities. He may express frustration and a sense of boredom when at home, particularly if some previous activities, such as going for walks, are no longer possible. He may also spend periods of time alone when members of his family are at work. These occasions may be especially hard if he misses the challenge and companionship of work. Thus, an actual problem in this AL may be recorded.

Planning care

Once sufficient information has been gathered and actual and potential patient problems have been documented, realistic and achievable goals can be set. These should be agreed with the patient whenever possible as this enhances the individuality of the planned care and improves the likelihood of goals being realistic. The use of both short-term and long-term goals is advocated by the model, measurable or observable patient outcomes being identified whenever this is feasible, together with an anticipated time span for the achievement of the goal.

Roper *et al.* acknowledge the importance of taking the availability of resources into account at this stage in the nursing process so that unrealistic expectations are not raised. This will be a familiar dilemma for many nurses when the resources required to give high-quality care are not always readily available. There is a considerable tension between not wanting to plan care that cannot be adequately resourced and embarking on a plan of care that does not offer the best that could be achieved if there were, for example, more qualified nursing staff or more equipment.

In the first example, problems related to dying alone and to expressing sexuality were noted. In addition, a disturbance to the woman's usual sleeping activity was identified. Goals set should solve or alleviate actual problems whenever possible and should aim to avoid potential problems becoming actual ones.

The ability to set a realistic goal related to the fear of dying provides an excellent example of the difficulty of setting goals without patient involvement. The nurse will need to be guided by the bereaved woman on what is likely to be achieved. It may be that death has always engendered feelings of apprehension, and the woman may be content with a short-term goal that focuses on identifying someone to talk to in the immediate period following her husband's death. A more long-term objective might relate to changes in her feelings about death.

A goal related to the tenth AL may be for the woman to feel that other ways of expressing her sexuality are an acceptable substitute for the physical contact she enjoyed with her husband. Alternatively, she may want to be able to talk to other members of her family or to particular friends about her need for physical touch, such as hugs, from those of whom she is fond.

With regard to sleep, goals may be set for the woman to achieve a certain number of hours sleep per night and for her to express less concern at her sleep pattern. Some problems cannot be solved but may be alleviated. It is likely that she will continue to dream about her husband, so a goal may be set related to a decrease in the emotional disturbance caused by the dreams.

For the man admitted for respite care and experiencing transient lower limb weakness, an actual problem with mobilising while an inpatient was identified, together with a potential problem of summoning family help at home to ensure his safety. In addition, he expressed feelings of boredom during times alone at home, with an associated sense of loss of the benefits derived from work and the work environment.

During a short inpatient stay such as that associated with respite care, it would be unrealistic to markedly alter the environment of care. Consequently, a goal may be set that focuses on the man's willingness to accept additional nursing assistance with mobility for the duration of his stay. Liaison with other professionals such as physiotherapists is entirely appropriate with the R–L–T model of nursing, and their involvement may be crucial to meeting an additional goal to maintain the man's mobility skills even with the restrictions of the inpatient environment.

The other two problems can be addressed during the inpatient stay but relate more closely to discharge planning. Assessment may have reassured the nurse and patient that he is able to identify when help is required for maintaining his safety and that he can use the hospital system for summoning help. However, a goal may be set to achieve a more satisfactory system for obtaining help when at home. The patient may have particular wishes about the activity of working and playing, and careful negotiation, perhaps involving an occupational therapist, will be needed to ensure that realistic and achievable goals are set in relation to the development of new pursuits. A further assessment in his own home may be required to establish what creative and challenging activities are feasible and affordable.

Finally, according to Roper *et al.* (1996), this stage is also the time for documenting the planned interventions to be carried out by the nurse and the patient in order for the goals to be achieved.

Nursing intervention and the delivery of care

The R–L–T model says little overtly about the principles that should guide nursing intervention, and this detracts from the model's utility. Indeed, despite their statement recognising the importance of nurses' decision-making being more explicit, the authors also claim:

Traditionally, nursing has been associated with 'doing', so nurses have little difficulty in knowing how to go about this phase of the process. (Roper *et al.*, 1996: 58)

It is hard to see how these two views can be compatible, and more guidance on ways of intervening and the skills required to successfully help patients achieve their goals would strengthen the model's appeal. This is particularly necessary when the authors claim that their model has particular usefulness for the neophyte student of nursing.

Certainly, no model can be comprehensive in its detail about nursing interventions, and current literature should always be an important source for evidence-based practice. What the model has to say about the nature of people does, however, offer some guidance. Using this model, nurses will sometimes intervene in ways that help people to maintain or regain independence in their ALs. Some nursing actions, therefore, may focus on teaching new skills. Similarly, the model sees the activity of communicating as important, and nurses themselves will need to be skilled communicators.

To return to the woman whose husband has died, the hospice nurse may be in a good position to talk with the woman about her fears related to death and dying. If a trusting relationship was established when the husband was being cared for, the woman may be more able to voice her concerns than with someone new. Hopefully, the care given to the husband might act as a starting point for discussion, explanations being offered for anything not well understood. It may be that the quality of the care given will help to allay the woman's fears. The nurse may also be able to help directly with the problem concerned with expressing sexuality by making time for discussion and by facilitating the involvement of relatives and/or friends. Sensitive subjects can sometimes be introduced by a nurse in such a way that other individuals can then continue to talk with less embarrassment.

Roper *et al.* suggest that some nursing activities can derive from medical instructions. Indeed, their published proforma for a care plan (Roper *et al.*, 1996) has a separate section for the recording of nursing interventions associated with medical (or other) prescription(s). For the recently bereaved woman, the nurse may thus work in collaboration with the woman's GP to ensure that, in the short term, she has a suitable night sedation prescribed to ensure that her goal for sleeping is met.

It is not uncommon for those recently bereaved to be disturbed by dreams, and reassurance that this is a recognised, if troubling, feature of bereavement may go some way to lessening the emotional upset caused. Furthermore, recognising that such dreams are not unusual may enable the woman to talk about them more easily with her friends and family. In this way, she may derive additional reassurance and be able to cope with them better.

Involving others in the interventions planned for the man with limb weakness may also maximise the likelihood of the set goals being achieved. In order to preserve his mobility skills, he may benefit from the assistance of a physiotherapist, who may be able to devise different ways of helping him to walk about and may take him to the gym for particular practice opportunities.

In relation to maintaining a safe environment, his family carers may need to leave him for periods of time at home. They might all benefit from the provision of a mobile telephone and/or some kind of medical alert device. This could both enhance the man's safety and enable his family carers to meet their own needs in relation to working and playing (AL 9). To achieve this, family members may need suitable local information about how such aids to independence can be acquired.

Given the transient and therefore variable nature of the lower limb weakness, a range of suitable pursuits may be the ideal for this man. The nurse could enlist the specialist skills of an occupational therapist, and together they might make suggestions about possible activities and if necessary develop a teaching programme for any new skills needed. The model's emphasis on maintaining usual activities suggests that attention should be paid to the man's previous interests rather than introducing something totally novel.

In an effort to compensate for the lack of social contact often experienced by those who spend prolonged periods at home, opportunities might be explored for the man to join a local association related to a realistic leisure activity of his choice.

Evaluation

The starting point for evaluation should be the goals originally set during the planning of nursing care. Following a specified period of nursing intervention, each AL should be re-examined to establish whether or not the goal set has been achieved. Roper *et al.* (1996) have identified the particularly complex nature of evaluation in nursing. Even if, for example, a goal has been met in the desired time frame, questions still remain. The goal set might have been too modest for the patient's potential abilities, and the achievement of a goal can rarely be easily explained given the interpendence of the contributions made by the patient, the nurse, family members and other health professionals.

Thus, the hospice nurse may quite soon be able to evaluate the success or otherwise of measures to ensure that the bereaved woman gets adequate sleep. Similarly, in the short term, it may be possible to achieve the goal of identifying people suitable for her to talk to about her fear of dying, expressing her sexuality and the troublesome dreams. Rather longer will be needed, for example, to know whether her fear of dying has been alleviated. This will probably be evaluated through the woman's expesed feelings.

The evaluation of the achievement of goals for the man with lower limb weakness will also take place over a span of time. Goals related to his inpatient care, such as accepting nursing help to walk about, may be evaluated early on in his stay. In the longer term, evaluation that his mobility skills were not compromised while in respite care may involve liaison with him after discharge. Similarly, it may only be after a period of time at home that it will be clear whether he is more content with his activities related to working and playing, and whether he has acquired an improved method of summoning help to ensure his safety.

Summative evaluation of the R–L–T model of nursing should involve an exploration of the extent to which it seems able to provide sensitive and appropriate standards of nursing within a given speciality or area of care. Over time, therefore, nurses working together should try to assess the contribution that the model makes to their practice. Some nursing models focus more overtly on people's psychological and social needs. It is important to consider the way in which this model advocates understanding the needs of individuals, primarily through a detailed assessment of their physical abilities and the impact of various influencing factors. In addition, nurses may wish to explore the extent to which this model assigns them a role in patient care different from that provided by doctors and other health care personnel.

References

Erickson, E. (1950) *Childhood and Society*. New York, Norton.

Maslow, A.H. (1954) *Motivation and Personality*. New York, Harper & Row.

Newton, C. (1991) *The Roper–Logan–Tierney Model in Action*. Basingstoke, Macmillan Press.

Roper, N. (1976) *Clinical Experience in Nurse Education*. Edinburgh, Churchill Livingstone.

Roper, N., Logan, W. and Tierney, A. (1980) *The Elements of Nursing*. Edinburgh, Churchill Livingstone.

Roper, N., Logan, W. and Tierney, A. (1981) *Learning to Use the Process of Nursing*. Edinburgh, Churchill Livingstone.

Roper, N., Logan, W. and Tierney, A. (1983) *Using a Model for Nursing*. Edinburgh, Churchill Livingstone.

Roper, N., Logan, W. and Tierney, A. (1985) *The Elements of Nursing*, 2nd edn. Edinburgh, Churchill Livingstone.

Roper, N., Logan, W. and Tierney, A. (1996) *The Elements of Nursing*, 4th edn. Edinburgh, Churchill Livingstone.

Wilson-Barnett, J. (1981) Book review. *Journal of Advanced Nursing*, 6, 249.

Chapter 6 Johnson's behavioural systems model of nursing

Both Henderson's and Roper *et al.*'s models of nursing see human behaviour as the outcome of an interaction between biological, psychological and social factors. Both tend to accept the validity of the medical model as a way of explaining the causes of ill-health but seek to add new dimensions to it – fundamental human needs in the case of Henderson, and ALs in the case of Roper *et al.* – when it comes to understanding nursing care. The model of nursing described in this chapter is, however, more radical in its nature and encourages us to focus on the behaviours that people display rather than upon their needs as such. This is why it is called the behavioural systems model of nursing.

Its developer, Dorothy Johnson, was a well-known nurse educator who worked at the University of California in Los Angeles between 1949 and 1978. Interestingly, while Johnson talked about aspects of her model on several occasions (for example Johnson 1968, 1978), and influenced others to write about it (for example Grubbs, 1974; Augur, 1976), it was not until after her retirement that she prepared the first full description of it for publication (Johnson, 1980). In the interim, she had written many other papers. In one of these, 'The nature of science in nursing', she distinguishes between the knowledge provided by the natural and applied sciences, and the knowledge that could be generated through nursing science (Johnson, 1959). The latter included knowledge acquired through observing the predictable responses that occur following patterns of nursing intervention. In a second paper, entitled 'Development of theory: a requisite for nursing as a primary health profession', she argued that a distinctive knowledge base was a prerequisite for nursing becoming a profession (Johnson,1974). Work to develop conceptual models of nursing was part of the process by which this knowledge could be generated.

Key components of care

The nature of people

From early in her work, Johnson was interested in how people respond biologically, psychologically, behaviourally and socially to stress, and this interest encouraged her to see individuals as having a set of interrelated behavioural subsystems, each striving for balance and equilibrium within itself. Seven major subsystems are identified – the affiliative, the achievement, the aggressive, the dependency, the eliminative, the ingestive and the sexual subsystems (Johnson, 1980, 1990). Each of these subsystems motivates behaviour towards the attainment of certain goals, as shown in Table 6.1. If one or more of these systems is in disequilibrium, less energy is likely to be available for recovery.

Table 6.1 Johnson's seven behavioural subsystems and the goals towards which they motivate behaviour

Subsystem	Behaviour motivated
Achievement	Towards control over oneself and one's environment
Affiliative	Towards relationships of intimacy with others
Aggressive	Towards self-protection from threat and towards self-assertion
Dependency	Towards conditions of security and dependency on others
Eliminative	Towards the expulsion of biological waste
Ingestive	Towards maintaining the integrity of the organism and towards achieving states of bodily pleasure
Sexual	Towards sexual gratification and towards caring for others

The action of each subsystem is, however, limited by a number of factors. These include past experience, people's perceptions of the behavioural options open to them, and people's understandings of what they can and cannot do. Some of these factors are what are called *sets* and arise through maturation, experience and learning. Two different kinds of set can be identified: *perseverative sets* created by past habits, and *preparatory sets*, which arise in response to the actions and objects immediately around a person. Further limitations on the actions of subsystems arise from people's *choices*, and these must sometimes be modified if subsystems in disequilibrium are to be restored to balance.

Underpinning many of Johnson's ideas about people are theoretical insights derived from research on drives and motivations (for example Hull, 1956), responses to stress and growth, self-actualisation and development (for example Maslow, 1970; Rogers, 1951). Also evident is a recognition of the self as being constituted through past experience and learning, a view much in keeping with the work of social learning theorists such as Bandura (1969). Johnson drew eclectically upon these insights and others in her effort to develop a model of nursing that would contribute to nursing knowledge and science, and to nursing's broader claims to being a profession.

The causes of problems likely to require nursing intervention

According to Johnson's model of nursing, behavioural subsystems can be thrown into disequilibrium by processes associated with disease or by processes linked to changes in personal requirements or patterns of daily living. Two kinds of disequilibrium can be envisaged: *internal subsystem problems*, and *intersystem problems*, which arise when one or more subsystems dominate the entire system. In either case, it is the nurses's responsibility to help disturbed subsystems to regain a state of balance. This can only be carried out once a nursing assessment has taken place.

The nature of assessment

Nursing assessment should be neither haphazard nor intuitive but should seek to generate empirical knowledge about behavioural subsystems and their state of balance or equilibrium. Ideally, assessment should proceed by examining each subsystem in turn to identify balance or imbalance within it. An assessment of the overall balance that exists between systems can then be carried out. According to Grubbs (1980), assessment may take place in two stages. First, subsystems are examined in turn to detect those which are out of equilibrium. Second, possible causes of imbalance are identified.

The nature of planning and goal-setting

A care plan is then drawn up by the nurse, based on each subsystem examined and on knowledge about the overall state of balance that exists between subsystems. Nurses should aim to intervene in order to provide the *sustenal imperatives* essential for balance to be restored within (and perhaps between) subsystems. *Protection, nurturance* and *stimulation* are among the techniques available to the nurse in restoring equilibrium, and environmental variables are likely to require manipulation in order to bring about the desired effects. Very little is said about the involvement of the care-receiver in planning and goal-setting using this model, a point to which we will return later.

The focus of nursing intervention during implementation of the care plan

Nursing intervention can take place in one of four ways using this model:

1. Nurses may *restrict* behaviours by imposing external constraints and controls.
2. Nurses may *defend* the individual by offering protection against external stressors and threats.
3. Nurses may attempt to *inhibit* the person by suppressing ineffective responses.
4. Nurses may *facilitate* the person by offering nurturance and stimulation.

These rather controlling behaviours on the part of the nurse are central to this model and its application.

The nature of evaluation

Evaluation requires the setting of long-term, intermediate and short-term goals for each person receiving nursing care. These goals must be related to specific subsystems and specified in observable and behavioural terms. Once this has been done, it will be possible to see whether they have been attained at the end of a designated period of time. This kind of ongoing or formative evaluation is, of course, different from the summative evaluation needed to decide whether the model is appropriate for use within a particular setting or context. For the latter to take place, nurses will need to consider whether the principles and commitments of the model match those found valuable within the area of care.

The role of the nurse

For Johnson (1992: 26–7), the social mission of nursing lies in its capacity to promote:

the most effective and efficient behavioural system possible, as well as to prevent specific problems from occurring in the system. Meeting this responsibility would also contribute to healthier biologic and social systems.

The nursing role is seen as complementary to that of the doctor but not dependent upon it. Nursing's distinctive contribution to care is through the imposition of control mechanisms that facilitate optimal levels of behaviour by restoring balance within or between affected subsystems. A preventive role for the nurse is also foreseen by the model, which advocates that nurses should have a role to play in anticipating the kinds of subsystem imbalance that could lead to later problems.

Using Johnson's model

Unlike the models considered so far, Johnson's model places particular emphasis on people's behaviour, which is viewed as 'patterned, repetitive, and purposeful' (Johnson, 1980: 209). As we have seen, Johnson identified seven major and interdependent behavioural subsystems. While the model draws many of its ideas from humanistic understandings that advocate holistic approaches to people, an examination of each subsystem is seen as an appropriate way of determining a person's functioning. This is because the whole system is dependent on each subsystem for its functional capacity. In this chapter, two examples of the model in practice will be discussed.

The first example focuses on an elderly man attending a hospital outpatients department who is found to have a possible problem in the ingestive subsystem. The other example considers a woman seeking advice and help in relation to the sexual subsystem. What these examples aim to do is to show how Johnson's model can offer an alternative to the more medically influenced models described in earlier chapters.

Assessment

Johnson's model requires a two-stage assessment process. Initially, the nurse carries out a careful examination of each subsystem to determine whether or not it is in balance. Such assessment will look particularly at observable behaviour and will also include reports by the patient on his or her behavioural tendencies and habits. There may be times when information will be sought from concerned relatives or friends so that as complete a picture as possible is built up. The first stage culminates in identifying the subsystem or subsystems in disequilibrium. The next stage seeks further information about the patient so that the cause of any lack of balance can be identified.

Assessment – first stage

According to Johnson, nursing assessment should be neither haphazard nor intuitive. Instead, it needs to be organised around a careful examination of each behavioural subsystem in turn, the nurse aiming to identify any evidence of relative balance or imbalance within each. The nurse can then begin to ascertain whether her role will be one of fostering effective behaviour or attempting to change behaviour that is not sufficiently supportive to the individual's overall functioning.

The elderly man attending for an outpatient appointment may be concerned at his unplanned weight loss over several months. At first sight, an imbalance might be suspected within the ingestive subsystem, and the nurse is therefore likely to focus her attention on this subsystem to begin with. She will probably weigh the man and measure his height in order to calculate his Body Mass Index, currently seen as a useful and simple indicator of nutritional status (Webb, 1995). Johnson describes and advocates both the science and the art of nursing, so carrying out measurements and developing insights and understandings all have a place within the assessment process. The nurse will be interested to know what weight the man used to be, and she will observe for outward signs of weight loss such as ill-fitting clothes, loose skin and poorly fitting dentures.

Although it may appear that the chief problem is located within the ingestive subsystem, the nurse will also consider the other subsystems to ascertain whether behaviour relating to these is contributing to the weight loss. Through careful questioning, she may discover that the man was bereaved several months ago and is now living alone and trying to cope with everyday chores with which he is unfamiliar. Imbalances may be found, therefore, in the achievement subsystem, where the man may be struggling with what Johnson tentatively calls 'caretaking skills' (Johnson, 1980: 214), and in the dependency and affiliative subsystems, where he may be missing his previous intimacy with his wife but may not have developed other social contacts. George (1995), among others, supports the need for assessment questions related to the affiliative subsystem to consider the individual's social system and the presence or absence of a significant other.

In the second example, a woman and her partner may have been referred to an infertility clinic following difficulties in conceiving. To begin with, the first stage assessment may concentrate on the sexual subsystem, with its dual functions of procreation and gratification. Johnson sees the sexual subsystem as having 'strong biologic system connotations' (Johnson, 1980: 213) as well as behaviours that are influenced by learning and cultural expectations.

First-stage assessment in this instance may take some considerable time and may extend over more than one visit because the issues involved are ones of an intimate and complex nature. The nurse may discover that the acknowledged disequilibrium in the sexual subsystem is accompanied by the potential for even greater imbalance in the affiliative subsystem if the woman's need for a baby and the establishment of a strong mother–child bond is, for her, a significant subsystem goal.

Assessment – second stage

During the second stage of assessment, a more detailed examination of those subsystems already identified as out of balance is carried out, with the goal of discovering the probable cause(s) of the disequilibrium. Johnson argues that problems arise when there are disturbances in either subsystem *structure* or subsystem *function*. As modes of intervention vary according to the type of problem, it is important during this second stage that the nurse can identify any difficulties as being structural or functional. In essence, structural problems arise within the subsystem itself while functional problems arise more from factors in the external environment.

In the case of the elderly man, the nurse may spend time asking him about what he eats and how he feels about eating food when it is prepared. She may find out whether he feels any discomfort when eating or after taking food. Critically, she may be interested in any variation in appetite or pleasure in food when meals are prepared by someone else or eaten in the company of others. The data she gathers may confirm that the ingestive subsystem is structurally intact but that its function is influenced by factors in the external environment, such as a lack of social contact, and limited by difficulties in other subsystems. In other words, the man may be able to eat with no discomfort or problem but his meals may be nutritionally poor and he may frequently lack the motivation to prepare meals or to eat enough for his bodily needs.

In this instance, the strength of the *drive* to prepare an adequate diet may be very weak in the achievement subsystem. Added to this may be the *limited range of behaviours* available to the man to complete household tasks and a tendency to act in particular ways (set), which reflect his greater familiarity with living with someone else rather than on his own. There may be structural problems in the dependency subsystem, the man's range of behaviours proving inadequate for him to gain attention, recognition and approval from others. There may also be reduced motivation (drive) in the affiliative subsystem to maintain or build relationships. Such difficulties are not uncommon when someone is bereaved and suffering a grief reaction (Sidell, 1993).

The sexual subsystem incorporates behaviours that are both biological and social. For the woman attending the infertility clinic, the biological functioning of the subsystem is her major problem. The level of behavioural functioning of the subsystem is less than optimal, and the subsystem is failing to achieve one of its goals, that of procreation. The nurse may work closely with medical colleagues to support the woman and her partner through the various tests and examinations that may be necessary to establish in more detail the likely cause of her inability to have a child.

Further assessment will also, however, concentrate on the woman's concerns about her need for a baby in order to meet the goal (drive) of her affiliative subsystem. Within any subsystem, the drive may be much stronger in some individuals than in others, and the nurse may discover that the woman values highly her drive to establish the mother–child bond. Both the nurse and the woman herself may see this as a potential future problem if she does not ultimately have a child. The nurse may also note that the woman's sense of personal worth is under threat (aggressive subsystem). Considerable uncertainty exists concerning the success of interventions to achieve a viable pregnancy in couples having fertility problems (Flores, 1996). The nurse may, therefore, want to continue an exploration of the wider personal issues confronting the woman. These concerns may indeed be the area of greatest import for the woman in her discussions with the nurse, whereas biological difficulties may dominate the patient–doctor relationship.

During the assessment process, the nurse will also need to be alert to any information that might be forthcoming about what Johnson calls 'sustenal imperatives'. According to Johnson:

The biologic system and all other living systems have the same requirements. Each must be *protected... nurtured...* and *stimulated...* to enhance growth and prevent stagnation. (1980: 212)

It is frequently in the areas of protection, nurturance and stimulation that nurses will be able to intervene to effect positive behavioural change. The elderly man may be receiving inadequate nurturance and stimulation, whereas the woman may be overstimulated by high hopes of treatment success.

Planning care

Once nursing problems have been identified, the nurse devises a care plan. Johnson's model sees the goal of nursing activities as restoring, maintaining or attaining behavioural system stability or homeostasis at the highest achievable level for the patient concerned. It says relatively little, however, about patient involvement in goal-setting, which can make planning for implementation difficult (George, 1995).

Johnson regards nurses as providers of an external *regulatory force* that 'operates through the imposition of external regulatory or control mechanisms' (Johnson, 1980: 214). The language selected by Johnson to describe the nursing role fits somewhat uneasily with current concerns emphasising the value of partnership and mutual regard between health workers and consumers of health care. The words 'regulatory force' suggest a relationship of considerable inequality, and nurses considering working with Johnson's model will therefore need to examine its main premises with care (Fraser, 1996). The emphasis on control strategies directed toward behavioural change may not always seem appropriate in care settings. There are, however, advocates for behavioural approaches in health care, often including systems of reward and punishment, when behaviour is considered inappropriate or maladaptive, or when someone's social skill repertoire is regarded as being limited (for example Hume, 1990; Milne, 1993).

Although Johnson's model includes references to similarly controlling interventions, it can be modified by including care practices more favourable to equality between nurses and patients, and by encouraging patient participation. Thus, planning care with this model may be improved by nurses jointly setting goals with patients. For example, a plan that establishes a goal of weight gain and better eating habits for the elderly man but which fails to take into account what he believes can be realistically achieved will probably fail. Together, the nurse and patient may decide that a long-term goal of reaching a particular weight is dependent on achieving certain other short-term goals. A goal may be agreed for him to learn to prepare foods that he likes, that are within his price range and that are relatively simple to make. A subsequent goal may focus more on his knowledge of suitable foods to make up a balanced diet. Another short-term goal may be to investigate acceptable ways for him to develop new social contacts.

At assessment, the drive to prepare food was thought to be lacking. An educational approach that extends his behavioural repertoire might mean that demonstrating new skills becomes an important drive in itself, with the added benefit of meals prepared. The nurse may also seek the man's view about learning within a group so that opportunities may be provided for him to learn alongside others, thus helping with the need for social contact.

In the second example, much of the planning in relation to goals in the biological part of the woman's sexual subsystem may be carried out by medical staff with the woman and her partner. Johnson sees nursing as being complementary to medicine but not dependent on it. Nursing attention may be more directed towards planning support for the woman while medical investigations and interventions take place.

Goals could be set in relation to the woman's aggressive subsystem. Johnson points out that, in her model, the aggressive subsystem is not concerned with the intent to injure others but is instead focused on the self, including the preservation of self-respect and personal control (Johnson, 1980). Goals might be agreed that aim for the woman to be empowered by the nurse, possibly acting in an advocacy role, to seek information from her doctors that will enable her to take part as an equal in decisions about her care. Another goal might be concerned with the woman gaining detailed knowledge of the planned medical procedures so that she feels in control while they take place. Knowing the success rates of infertility treatment, the nurse will hope that adequate planning in the aggressive subsystem will avoid any further feelings of lack of self-respect for the woman if medical treatment for herself and/or her partner proves unsuccessful.

Assessment also identified concerns within the affiliative subsystem. Goals in this area may be difficult to set as the woman's attention (drive) will be highly focused on the biological functioning of the sexual subsystem. Together, the woman and the nurse may agree that the only realistic short-term goal is one that aims for a designated time for discussion about the woman's needs in the affiliative subsystem, with a longer-term goal of exploring how her needs might be met through other relationships with her family or friends. High and sometimes unrealistic hopes of a successful outcome from medical treatment may cause some ambivalence from the woman about the need for such discussion and goals. However, a recognition that the perceived value of these goals may change as medical interventions progress may help to establish the ongoing and dynamic nature of the nurse–patient relationship.

Nursing intervention and the delivery of care

According to Johnson, the major aim of nursing intervention is to ensure the fulfilment of the goals of each behavioural subsystem. There is a need for *protection* from influences with which the system cannot cope, *nurturance* in the form of various inputs from the environment and *stimulation* for growth. As stated earlier, nurses intervene in a variety of ways, specifically by *restricting* someone's behaviour, by *defending* someone from external stressors or threats, by *inhibiting* someone by helping them to suppress ineffective behaviour and finally by *facilitating* someone through nurturance and stimulation.

The elderly man has been bereaved, and the sustenal imperatives of nurturance and stimulation may have originated from his relationship with his wife. The goal of helping him to prepare more adequate meals might initially be met by the nurse in a facilitative role. The help of an occupational therapist could be valuable in teaching new skills. Then, if the nurse is able to offer outreach help, she might visit the man at home to be present when a meal is prepared so that positive feedback on his skills can be given. The nurturing of new behaviours should help to confirm for him that his range of behaviours in relation to preparing food has increased. A home visit may also stimulate him to see benefit in social contact at home and encourage him to invite friends to his house.

If the man feels able to attend a group activity in relation to nutrition and food preparation, this might be helpful. With an increasing number of elderly people living longer, day and evening classes have developed to meet their particular needs, and nurses may be able to stimulate particular events in their local community. Writing in the USA, Dodge and Knutesen (1994) advocate a community approach to nutritional problems for older people, including ongoing nutrition education classes as one strategy to promote a healthy diet. In Britain, nurses have traditionally intervened with individuals, couples or small groups, but there is a growing recognition of the value of trying to influence the wider community in relation to health issues (Ewles and Simnett, 1995).

Although bereavement and grief have played an important part in the man's difficulties, Johnson's model directs attention to interventions related to the behavioural outcomes of his grief rather than to the grief process itself. Its approach here is similar to that of behaviour therapy, which places less importance on the thoughts and feelings associated with behavioural change and more on strategies to encourage new behaviours. This is in marked contrast to, for example, a model such as Peplau's (see Chapter 10), in which the focus of intervention would be the grief reaction itself.

Nursing intervention for the woman will initially focus on helping her to understand the medical investigations and possible treatments in relation to infertility. In this way, the nurse can defend the woman from the undue stress often experienced when individuals feel that they lack control. There may be written leaflets available for the woman and her partner, and the nurse will be able to check the woman's understanding and answer any outstanding questions. Sometimes, the nurse will be able to put different patients in touch with each other for mutual support. Both the receiving and giving of support may help the woman to achieve the goal of the aggressive subsystem in that she may value her own contribution to someone else's well-being.

Gaining knowledge and understanding will go some way to meeting the goal of being empowered to discuss treatment decisions with the doctor. In addition, the nurse may provide opportunites for the woman to try out what she might say to her doctor in order to increase her confidence. This kind of facilitation by the nurse can stimulate the growth of new behaviours, in this case a more assertive approach to medical consultation. In Johnson's model, self-assertion is a recognised drive within the aggressive subsystem.

Achieving designated discussion time for the woman to explore her feelings about the affiliative subsystem's drive for her to conceive will require commitment from both the woman and the nurse. The nurse will need to ensure that a suitable environment is available for the discussion of issues of a very sensitive and personal nature. It may be difficult at first to encourage discussion that goes beyond the biological functioning of the sexual subsystem. A regulatory and controlling role may have to be taken on by the nurse in establishing ground rules with the woman about the need for the designated discussion times to focus on the affiliative subsystem.

Evaluation

Anticipated and desired outcomes of nursing intervention with Johnson's model will focus largely on observable and reported behaviour in relation to the goals set at the planning stage. As stated earlier, Johnson's view of nursing values both the science and the art of practice. The nurse will therefore look for specific evidence of goal achievement; where possible, this will be observed behaviour. Intuition is not advocated as a nursing skill in this model, so even when directly observable behaviour is not available, the nurse will need clear evidence of behavioural outcomes.

In the longer term, the evaluation of the success of nursing intervention for the elderly man will include measuring his weight and recalculating his Body Mass Index, as well as ascertaining through discussion whether his concern about his weight has passed. As is often the case in health care, however, the presenting problem of weight loss masks more important difficulties.

Thus, in the short term, the nurse will look for evidence of change in the achievement and affiliative subsystems. She will observe the man's ability to prepare meals effectively and ask him about healthy food choices. She may look for evidence in the man's behaviour and speech of an increased interest in caring for himself and in maintaining friendships. He may talk positively about a sense of achievement in learning new household skills. He may describe time spent in the company of others. A diary record might prove useful for him to report his meals and his social activities over a period of time. This not only provides evaluative material for the nurse, but may also serve as a motivator and positive reinforcer for the elderly man himself.

There will also be behaviour to observe directly in order to evaluate the success or otherwise of nursing interventions for the woman attending the infertility clinic. The nurse may witness discussions between the patient and doctor in which the woman demonstrates her knowledge of what is happening to her and in which she takes an active part in treatment decisions. Body language may also be a guide for the nurse in evaluating how confident the woman feels. Discussion between the woman and the nurse may provide opportunities for the nurse to ask how in control the woman feels and thus to assess growth in the aggressive subsystem.

Evaluation of development in the affiliative subsystem may be very tentative while more medical treatment options in relation to the biological functioning of the sexual subsystem are tried out. The reality may be that, for a long time, only the achievement of time for discussion can be judged. This can, however, provide reassurance for the woman that other personal issues have not been forgotten, and she and the nurse may agree that while the outcome of medical treatment remains uncertain, potential difficulties in the affiliative subsystem can be discussed but not addressed. As stated earlier, there must be a realism in planned nursing interventions that can only be achieved through a partnership approach to care.

Nurses who choose to work with Johnson's model will need to gather evaluative data over time from their contact with several patients whose main problems are demonstrated through their behaviour. They will need to decide whether the rather controlling nursing role advocated in the model is suitable for current health care, and if not, whether Johnson's model can be modified to offer a behavioural approach more sympathetic to patient participation. It is probable that there will always be occasions when the focus of this model will be particularly appropriate for someone's care. The challenge for nurses who are familiar with a number of models is to develop criteria that will facilitate the selection of the most suitable nursing model at a very early stage in the assessment process.

References

Augur, J.R. (1976) *Behavioral Systems and Nursing*. Englewood Cliffs, NJ, Prentice Hall.

Bandura, A. (1969) *Principles of Behavior Modification*. New York, Harper & Row.

Dodge, J. and Knutesen, P. (1994) Enhancing health and function in late life. In Webb, P. (ed.) *Health Promotion and Patient Education*. London, Chapman & Hall.

Ewles, L. and Simnett, I. (1995) *Promoting Health*. Chichester, John Wiley & Sons.

Flores, L.A. (1996) Options and risks with reproductive technologies. In Parrott, R.L. and Condit, C.M (eds) *Evaluating Women's Health Messages*. London, Sage.

Fraser, M. (1996) *Conceptual Nursing in Practice: A Research-Based Approach*. London, Chapman & Hall.

George, J.B. (1995) *Nursing Theories: The Base for Professional Nursing Practice*. London, Prentice Hall.

Grubbs, J. (1974) An interpretation of the Johnson behavioral systems model. In Riehl, J.P. and Roy, C. (eds) *Conceptual Models for Nursing Practice*. Norwalk, CT, Appleton-Century-Crofts.

Grubbs, J. (1980) An interpretation of the Johnson behavioral systems model. In Riehl, J.P and Roy, C. (eds) *Conceptual Models for Nursing Practice*, 2nd edn. Norwalk, CT, Appleton-Century-Crofts.

Hull, C.L. (1956) *Essentials of Behaviour*. New Haven, Yale University Press.

Hume, A. (1990) Behaviour therapy model: principles and general applications. In Reynolds, W. and Cormack, D. (eds) *Psychiatric and Mental Health Nursing: Theory and Practice*. London, Chapman & Hall.

Johnson, D.E. (1959) The nature of a science of nursing. *Nursing Outlook*, 7(5): 291–4.

Johnson, D.E. (1968) One Conceptual Model of Nursing. Paper presented at Vanderbildt University, Nashville, TN, April.

Johnson, D.E. (1974) Development of theory: a requisite for nursing as a primary health profession. *Nursing Outlook*, 23(5): 372–7.

Johnson, D.E. (1978) Behavioral System Model for Nursing. Paper presented at the Second Annual Nurse Educator Conference, New York (Cassette Recording), December.

Johnson, D.E. (1980) The behavioral system model for nursing. In Riehl, J.P. and Roy, C. (eds) *Conceptual Models for Nursing Practice*, 2nd edn. Norwalk, CT, Appleton-Century-Crofts.

Johnson, D.E. (1990) The behavioral system model for nursing. In. Parker, M.E (ed.) *Nursing Theories in Practice*. New York, National League for Nursing.

Johnson, D.E. (1992) The origins of the behavioral system model. In Nightingale, F.N. *Notes on Nursing: What It Is, What It Is Not* (Commemorative edition). Philadelphia, PA, J.B. Lippincott.

Maslow, A. (1970) *Motivation and Personality*. New York, Harper & Row.

Milne, D. (1993) *Psychology and Mental Health Nursing*. London, Macmillan.

Rogers, C. (1951) *Client-centred Therapy*. Boston, Houghton-Mifflin.

Sidell, M. (1993) Death, dying and bereavement. In Bond, J., Coleman, P. and Peace, S. (eds) *Ageing in Society*. London, Sage.

Webb, G.P. (1995) *Nutrition – a Health Promotion Approach*. London, Edward Arnold.

Chapter 7 Roy's adaptation model of nursing

One of the best known models of nursing is the Roy adaptation model (RAM). Developed by Callista Roy, a member of the Sisters of Saint Joseph of Carondelet, the model has stimulated nurse researchers, nurse educators and practising nurses world wide. Why this should be so we will explore further in this chapter. We will begin, however, by saying a little about Roy herself. After receiving her initial qualification in nursing from Mount Saint Mary's College in Los Angeles, Roy went on to gain further qualifications in both nursing and sociology from the University of California, Los Angeles. She was stimulated to develop her model of nursing when challenged to do so in a seminar by Dorothy Johnson (see Chapter 6), and oversaw its initial use as the philosophical basis of the nursing curriculum at Mount Saint Mary's College where she later taught. She has written numerous books including *Introduction to Nursing: An Adaptation Model* (Roy, 1976; 2nd edition, 1984), *Theory Construction in Nursing: An Adaptation Model* (Roy and Roberts, 1981) and *The Roy Adaptation Model: The Definitive Statement* (Roy and Andrews, 1991). In 1988, she took up a senior position at Boston College School of Nursing in Massachusetts.

Roy's intellectual development was much influenced by systems theory (von Bertalanffy, 1968) and by Helson's (1964) adaptation theory, both of which she encountered in the course of her postgraduate studies. From systems theory, she developed the idea that people are best characterised by holism, interdependence, control processes, information feedback and complexity. From adaptation theory, she took the ideas that human behaviour is essentially adaptive, and that adaptation levels vary between people depending on circumstances. The philosophical underpinning of her model is broadly humanistic – people act purposefully and creatively, need relationships and are best characterised as integrated 'wholes'. They are:

adaptive system(s) constantly growing and developing within a changing environment. A person's health can be described as a reflection of this interaction or adaptation. (Andrews and Roy, 1991: 19)

Because of the emphasis on adaptation, the model is usually referred to as the Roy adaptation model of nursing.

Key components of care

The nature of people

Roy's model of nursing characterises people in terms very different from those with which we may be familiar. Roy says that humans are wholes in the sense that individual aspects of the person act together to form a unified being, but people comprise a number of interrelated systems. Three principal systems make up each person, but each is related to the others. These are the biological, psychological and social systems. Each system is in a state of constant interaction, both with other systems and with the environment. Systems cannot be looked at, like parts of the body, but their actions can be observed in individuals' behaviour and in their responses to disease, ill-health and nursing care.

According to Roy, each system strives for stability within itself, in its relationship to other systems and with the broader environment. There is nothing new in this idea, at least in relation to the idea of physiological balance, and the concept of homeostasis will be familiar to the majority of nurses. Where the RAM is innovative is in its suggestion that there exist within each of us forces towards *psychological* and *social* balance as well. Roy took these ideas from the work of Helson, who had suggested that there exists both physiological and behavioural homeostasis within the person. While the former enables balance in physiological systems such as those governing fluid balance and food intake, the latter helps people to cope with psychological and social experiences. Psychological and social systems also strive to maintain equilibrium and balance, since when they are balanced, people can deal best with their environmental experience and their relationships with one another. Psychological and social systems may affect physiological systems (and vice versa), implying the interrelatedness and holism that the RAM says is characteristic of us all.

It is important to emphasise, however, that there is no one 'perfect' state of balance applicable to everyone: people vary widely in the equilibria they seek to attain. It is important, therefore, for the nurse to recognise and work with the individuality of each person. Individuals strive to maintain their physiological, psychological and social systems within a range of conditions unique to themselves. According to Roy, such a set of conditions makes up a person's *adaptation level*. New stimuli that fall within this level of adaptation are likely to be responded to more favourably than those which fall outside it. Adaptation level is therefore little more than a range of adaptability within which it is possible to deal effectively with new experiences. This can be seen diagrammatically in Figure 7.1.

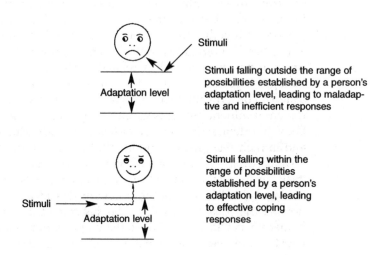

Figure 7.1   Adaptation level

The factors influencing a person's adaptation level are called stimuli. Three types of stimuli are particularly important in relation to the planning and provision of nursing care:

1. *Focal stimuli*, immediately surrounding a person
2. *Contextual stimuli*, linked to the context in which focal stimuli are present
3. *Residual stimuli*, such as beliefs, attitudes and values resulting from past patterns of learning.

In the health care setting, focal stimuli can include nurses, doctors and other health care personnel as well as the equipment and materials used to deliver care. Contextual stimuli, on the other hand, can include such variables as temperature and noise, which may occur alongside other more immediate sources of sensory stimulus. For many people, residual stimuli will derive from their previous experience, including that of health care such as visits to hospital, to the doctor or to the dentist.

Together, focal, contextual and residual stimuli establish the adaptation level characteristic of a person. This adaptation level in turn determines how the person responds to new stimuli. Two main types of response are possible:

1. *Adaptive responses*, which promote the integrity of the person, leading to growth, development and greater control over the environment among other consequences.
2. *Ineffective responses*, which do not lead to these outcomes.

The RAM identifies two other important subsystems within the individual, both associated with coping. The *regulator subsystem* is largely concerned with initiating and maintaining balance between (1) autonomic, (2) endocrine and (3) motor bodily responses. Roy explicitly identifies psychological as well as physiological factors contributing to each of these responses. The *cognator subsystem*, on the other hand, is largely concerned with attention and memory, learning, problem-solving and decision-making, and emotional attachments and defences. The two systems are interrelated, and outputs from the regulator system (bodily responses to tissue damage, for example) may be translated into perceptions (of pain) in the cognator system.

Although the existence of the regulator and cognator subsystems can be inferred from behaviour, neither is directly observable. Only the responses determined by these systems can be observed, measured or subjectively described. These responses can be of four main types or, as Roy puts it, can fall within one of four *adaptive modes*:

1. The physiological adaptive mode
2. The self-concept adaptive mode
3. The role-function adaptive mode
4. The interdependency adaptive mode.

Each of these modes contributes to the 'promotion of the adaptive goals of the total person system – survival, growth, reproduction and mastery' (Roy and McLeod, 1981: 67).

The physiological mode of adaptation is concerned largely with maintaining physiological balance with respect to oxygenation, nutrition, elimination, activity and rest, and protection against infection, including skin integrity. Physiological adaptation is largely influenced by the regulator subsystem.

The self-concept adaptive mode is concerned with the need for psychological integrity. It encompasses both the physical (or bodily) self and the personal self. Linked to the physical self is body image. Linked to the personal self are self-consistency, the self-ideal and the moral–ethical–spiritual self. People strive to maintain a balance between what they know is morally or ethically right, the kind of person they would like to be, and the person they know they are. Both the physical and the personal selves are interrelated, which has important implications for the ways in which nurses prepare patients for surgical procedures that may result in a changed sense of body image or physical self.

The third mode of adaptation – the role-function mode – is concerned with managing social interaction with others. It is linked to the attainment of social integrity. Three role functions are identified by the RAM. The primary role, linked principally to age, sex, social background and developmental stage, is the most enduring of the three. The secondary role is one that is achieved and relates to tasks that may need to be carried out at a particular developmental stage (for example those associated with being a pupil at school, having a particular job or being a parent). Tertiary roles are usually even more short lived and include the roles adopted when meeting obligations as well as hobbies. For acute illness, they can include the sick role (although for longer-term or terminal illness, the sick role may become secondary).

Finally, the interdependency mode is concerned with emotional and affective behaviour. Feelings of love, acceptance, rejection, hostility, rivalry, alienation and dominance are all controlled from within this mode. Friendliness, dominance and competitiveness are kinds of behaviour connected with this adaptive mode. Significant others and support systems are seen as the two major factors contributing to meeting interdependence needs.

Each of the above four modes of adaptation has important consequences for the planning and delivery of nursing care. Indeed, the specification of adaptive modes is reported as arising in response to requests from student nurses for greater guidance in organising assessment data. Difficulties within a particular mode can lead to the ineffective responses shown in Table 7.1.

Table 7.1   Modes of adaptation

Person	Problems within this mode can be associated with
Physiological adaptive mode	Hyperactivity, fatigue
	Malnutrition, vomiting
	Constipation, incontinence
	Oxygen deficit, oxygen excess
	Infection through the loss of skin integrity
Self-concept adaptive mode	Sense of physical loss
	Change of body image
	Sense of anxiety
	Sense of powerlessness
	Sense of low self-esteem
	Sense of inconsistency
Role-function adaptive mode	Sense of role failure
	Sense of role conflict
Interdependency adaptive mode	Sense of alienation
	Sense of rejection
	Sense of rivalry
	Sense of loneliness
	Sense of dominance

The causes of problems likely to require intervention

According to the RAM, nursing interventions are likely to be necessary when there is either a *need deficit* or a *need excess* within one or more of the four adaptive modes. Need deficits are usually associated with insufficiencies in the environmental resources available to a person with respect to one or more modes of adaptation. Need excesses are usually the result of an excess of environmental resources.

The nature of assessment

Roy advocates a three-stage assessment. In the first stage, and looking at each adaptive mode in turn, the nurse seeks to identify behaviours suggesting that coping mechanisms are strained. Assessment techniques can include direct observation, measurement using appropriate tools and tests, and interviewing to elicit subjective reports. Having identified such behaviours, the nurse must next decide whether the actions concerned are adaptive or ineffective. If they are of the former type, nursing intervention will aim to support them, whereas if they are of the latter variety, nursing intervention will seek to modify them.

A second-stage and more detailed assessment then takes place. This involves identifying specific focal, contextual and residual stimuli relating to the adaptation problems earlier identified. Second-stage assessment should involve the active participation of the patient, who may be called upon to validate (or otherwise) the stimuli that the nurse identifies as being particularly pertinent.

A third and final stage then ensues. Here, the nurse reaches a nursing diagnosis of the patient's adaptation status. This usually involves describing the behaviours indicative of poor adaptation within one or more modes and the stimuli that contribute to these behaviours. The nursing diagnosis forms the basis from which care planning can proceed.

The nature of planning and goal-setting

In the light of her assessment, the nurse should draw up with a patient a list of goals relating to the individual concerns. These should be placed in order of priority and should be written in patient-centred terms, specifying what the patient will be able to do when each goal has been achieved. A time frame should be attached to each goal, and it may be useful to distinguish between short-term and long-term goals when planning care. Goals should be stated both for ineffective behaviours that are to be changed and adaptive behaviours that may need reinforcement. Again, active patient involvement is advocated since someone who is actively involved in the formulation of goals is more likely to be committed to their attainment. As Roy and Roberts explain:

According to this nursing model, the person is to be respected as an active participant in his care... The goal arrived at is one of mutual agreement between nurses and patients. (1981: 47)

The focus of intervention during implementation of the care plan

According to the RAM, nursing interventions most usually involve manipulating focal and contextual stimuli in order to promote better adaptation within affected modes. Stimuli may be *altered, increased, decreased, removed* or *maintained* to do this. For maximum effectiveness, nurses will aim to intervene using stimuli that fall within a patient's present range of adaptation. This may involve, for example, using language and selecting nursing behaviours with which the person is already familiar. By the judicious manipulation of focal and contextual stimuli, the nurse will aim, where necessary, to modify present adaptation and coping.

The nature of evaluation

Evaluation involves examining whether each of the goals set during planning has been met. By doing this, the nurse can determine the extent to which adaptation within each affected mode has been strengthened. She will be hoping to find evidence of a greater number of adaptive responses and fewer ineffective ones. When goals are attained, they can be deleted from nursing concern; when they are not attained, reassessment is indicated, resulting perhaps in a redefinition of goals and/or a respecification of nursing interventions.

The role of the nurse

According to Roy and Roberts (1981), the nurse's role is to promote health in all life processes in the pursuit of 'higher level wellness'. In order to do this, much of the nurse's work aims to promote adaptive responses in each of the four adaptive modes. By manipulating focal and contextual stimuli, and by seeking to modify the influence of residual stimuli, nursing seeks to reduce ineffective responses and promote adaptive ones. The nurse's role is therefore broader than that of the doctor since it aims to promote patient adaptation in health and illness.

Using Roy's model

The central idea within the RAM is that people strive for equilibrium, or stability, within and between three systems (biological, psychological and social) and with the broader environment. Experienced nurses are likely to be attracted to this idea because people in health care situations frequently demonstrate the human capacity to adapt to significant physical and personal change. It is not unusual for nurses to comment on how well a patient copes with, for example, a major body image change or the resilience of family members to personal loss. Roy herself, when working as a paediatric nurse, 'had been impressed with the ability of children to bounce back when faced with illness' (cited in Lutjens, 1995: 95).

The two examples selected to illustrate the application of RAM to nursing practice focus on health-related responses primarily in the role-function and self-concept modes. One example considers a young gay man seeking specialist sexual health advice. The other explores body image changes for an adult woman who is in hospital receiving chemotherapy.

Assessment

As has been identified, throughout all three stages of assessment Roy advocates the need for a similar range of nursing skills, in particular those of careful and sensitive observation, accurate measurement and interviewing.

First stage – assessment of behaviour

Roy suggests that this early stage in the assessment process can be carried out fairly quickly in that it seeks to observe behaviour to determine whether there is a need for nursing and to tentatively identify which adaptive modes are under strain. According to Andrews and Roy (1991), the nurse should look systematically for observable behaviour in each of the four adaptive modes and should be alert to any additional non-observable behaviour. There is little detail in Roy's writings about assessing non-observable behaviour, but this is likely to focus on the person's reported feelings or concerns.

The young gay man arriving at a designated young person's health clinic is demonstrating adaptive behaviour that warrants support from the nurse. Attendance at the clinic shows insight into the need to gain information or help. This indicates effective activity within the cognator subsystem, and the nurse's response should emphasise its positive nature. Although Roy suggests that during this first stage, adaptive modes experiencing stress should be identified, this may not always happen. At this early stage, the nurse may only know that the man is seeking health advice and may not know which adaptive mode(s) is most affected.

Some progress has been made in Britain in helping to make young people feel more valued and welcome in health care settings, particularly those which attempt to address issues relevant to sexual health. The DoH issued guidance for health care professionals in 1993 in its *Key Area Handbook HIV/AIDS and Sexual Health*. Such guidance, including ways in which an atmosphere of positive regard can be engendered by paying attention to the physical environment and by respecting confidentiality, would find approval within the RAM because it seeks to support young people's adaptive behaviour.

In the second example, the hospital nurse may meet the patient prior to the commencement of chemotherapy and may observe through the patient's behaviour, perhaps her body language or her conversation, that the woman is worried. Even preliminary discussions can highlight key issues, and the woman may immediately express concerns about the expected hair loss as well as reservations about how she will cope with such a threat to her self-image. While acknowledging that this will not be the only problem, the nurse has ascertained something of particular importance to the patient and noted the strain on the self-concept mode.

Second stage – assessment of stimuli

During this second stage, a more detailed assessment is carried out to clarify which internal and external stimuli (known collectively by Roy as the 'environment') are most affecting the patient's behaviour. Both adaptive and ineffective behaviours identified during the first stage of assessment are important as the model seeks both to maintain adaptive behaviour and to change ineffective behaviour towards more adaptive responses.

According to Roy and Andrews (1991), it is knowledge of the stimuli that is crucial in enabling the nurse to help the patient to maintain or achieve adaptation. This is because the stimuli are seen as causative for the level of adaptation achieved. As each stimulus is identified, it is also classified as focal (sometimes called confronting), contextual or residual.

Within the literature on the RAM, there are many examples of what might constitute a particular stimulus. Rambo (1984), among others, argues that the focal stimulus will often stem from the diagnosed medical illness. While this may sometimes be the case, a focal stimulus may also be a critical personal event or crisis, or something significant in the immediate physical environment.

The role of residual stimuli in determining the adaptation level is open to debate. Some authors (for example Rambo, 1984; Lutjens, 1995) seem to suggest that, once recognised by a nurse, a residual stimulus must be recategorised. They argue that although residual stimuli are known to exist, they are not always confirmed during assessment, but if and when they are validated with and by the patient, they become contextual or even focal stimuli:

Residual stimuli are those general, vague, ambiguous factors that may be affecting a person, but their influence cannot be immediately ascertained or validated. After residual stimuli are validated, they become either focal or contextual stimuli. (Lutjens, 1995: 105–6)

Roy and Andrews (1991), however, continue to write of three separate types of stimulus and support the notion that the effect of residual stimuli may be indeterminate. They write of the value of the category of residual stimuli during assessment as providing a way for nurses to record their hunches or intuitive impressions about what might be affecting a person's adaptation level. They confirm that further assessment may change the category to contextual or focal but also state that recategorisation may occur in the other direction as well. Thus a focal stimulus, for example, may change to become residual.

This view of the nature of residual stimuli fits uneasily with the experience of many nurses who find that people's deeply held beliefs and attitudes are enduring and powerful influences on their health-related behaviours and especially on their decision-making in care settings. Such beliefs may be particularly challenging for a nurse to assess accurately, but this is not the same as saying they are vague or ambiguous. Nor does it seem likely that they will be 'just a possible influence' or in the background (Roy and Andrews, 1991: 10). We shall therefore continue to advocate the value of trying to determine which residual stimuli are contributing to a person's adaptation level and to advise against the need for always seeking to recategorise them as focal or contextual.

In the first example, the young man may be involved in a long-term sexual relationship with another man and may just have learned that a close friend is HIV positive. This may be the focal stimulus causing him to experience a degree of role conflict. Thus, on the one hand, he may view having sex with his partner as being essential to his own and his partner's well-being. On the other hand, he may be experiencing anxiety about the risks involved and therefore be seeking reassurance that his and his partner's current behaviour is as protective as possible. He may need such reassurance in order to fulfil his role as a sexually active gay man. He may feel some degree of role transition in that he has become a seeker of health advice, and he may acknowledge that some changes in his behaviour would constitute positive coping strategies as a response to his knowledge about HIV.

Contextual stimuli are those stimuli present within the context in which the focal stimulus has been found, or those stimuli which contribute to the impact of the focal stimulus. In this example, the young man's anxiety is influenced both by his knowledge of what being HIV positive may mean for his friend and by his concern about his friend's former partners. Coupled with this, he may have a strong sense of the need for people to take responsibility for their own health, particularly for the precautions necessary to avoid contracting or transmitting sexually transmitted diseases such as HIV. These concerns may form part of the residual stimuli (attitudes and beliefs) contributing to his adaptation level.

For the woman about to commence a course of chemotherapy, the strain on the self-concept mode may be influenced by her wish to continue with her job. She may be a counsellor offering a range of support services to others, both individually and in groups. Crucially, she may fear that her clients will be distracted from the purpose of their meetings if her appearance has markedly altered.

Thus, the focal stimulus may be the fear of a noticeable body image change, set against the contextual stimuli of the woman's job, her wish to continue to work and the particular needs of her client group. Added to this may be her belief that the relationship with her clients will be adversely affected if they observe her appearance to have changed. Such a belief may constitute a powerful residual stimulus.

In the second assessment stage, Roy advocates validating the information with the patient as far as possible. This can be done in a number of ways, particularly through corroborative data and patient comment. First, then, the nurse may seek corroboration from the data she gathers. She may look for consistencies in the information so that conclusions are not hastily drawn from single observations or measurements. This is an important step in validating assessment data as it provides a check that does not rely on the patient being able to comment verbally on ideas put to him. It should also mean that the nurse has reasonable confidence in her conclusions before asking the patient to validate them.

Third stage – nursing diagnosis

In the third stage, the nurse aims to formulate a nursing diagnosis from which a detailed plan of care can be developed. This diagnosis relies on a consideration of the information gathered at both the earlier stages of assessment. Details of Roy's typology of nursing diagnoses in each adaptive mode can be found in Roy and Andrews (1991).

The young man attending the health clinic is demonstrating an adaptive response in the role function mode to various influencing stimuli. He does this by showing what Roy and Andrews (1991: 39) describe as 'effective processes of role transition... effective processes for coping with role changes'. A nursing diagnosis that identifies positive life processes, as in this example, will generate a care plan that emphasises the nursing role of maintaining or enhancing adaptation.

In contrast, following the first two stages of assessment, the nurse may identify that, taken together, various stimuli are causing a significant strain on the woman's ability to adapt to the planned medical treatment. In the self-concept mode particularly, the nurse may diagnose anxiety about the personal self related to expected body image disturbance (physical self). She may also recognise that loss of contentment with her body image seems likely to disrupt the woman's confidence in her occupational role.

Planning care

With nursing diagnoses established, the nurse is in a position to generate a list of patient-centred goals. If at all possible, goals should be the product of discussion and agreement between the nurse and patient. This not only demonstrates that the nurse respects the patient's views, but also increases the chance of goals being achieved.

According to Roy and Andrews (1991), goals may be either short-term or long-term. Really short-term goals with a time frame of minutes or hours will usually only be appropriate in relation to critical, ineffective responses in the physiological adaptive mode. Goals will more often be set with longer time frames of days or even weeks.

A goal should identify the behaviour to be maintained or altered, the means of recognising whether the desired behaviour is happening and the time when goal achievement should occur. Usually, more than one goal will be established, and a priority order will be agreed.

The young man attending the sexual health clinic is demonstrating effective, adaptive behaviour in the role-function mode, which the nurse will wish to foster. She may, therefore, discuss with him a long-term goal that focuses on his continued willingness to seek appropriate sexual health advice for as long as he experiences anxiety about the precautions taken by him and his partner. Goal achievement may be recognised by his attendance at the clinic for a defined number of visits and eventually by his confidence to end his contact with the nurse. He may communicate this decision in person, over the telephone or in writing.

In the short term, goals might focus on the man's knowledge of the various modes of HIV transmission and on his understanding of the steps that gay men can take to protect against infection. Successful goal achievement might be measured by his ability to communicate his knowledge and understanding to the clinic nurse and by his reduced feelings of anxiety about his and his partner's risk of HIV.

The woman admitted to start a course of chemotherapy is demonstrating strain, particularly in the self-concept mode. Discussion between her and the nurse concerning goal-setting may involve a number of issues related to her response to the planned treatment. The nurse may first discuss the value to the woman of some up-to-date knowledge about both the degree of hair loss to be anticipated and the measures that can be taken to make the patient feel confident in her appearance. One short-term goal might therefore focus on a gain in knowledge. This may in itself enable the woman to feel more confident about her personal self-concept because having knowledge gives people more control over what is happening to them.

Evidence of goal achievement in this example might relate to the woman's expressed feelings of greater confidence. Depending on the other effects of her anxiety, in particular those mediated through the regulator subsystem, she might also demonstrate an improved sleep pattern or a reduction in blood pressure. Such a short-term goal might have a time frame of 1 day from admission as this time could well have been planned for information-giving and preparation prior to the commencement of medical treatment.

For the longer term, the nurse may advocate a goal related to the woman's fears about the impact of any change in her appearance on her relationship with clients. There could be value in revisiting the role and skills of a counsellor and in encouraging the patient to reflect on the positive rather than the negative changes that might result from her own health experience and subsequent empathy with her clients. Such a goal may take several days or weeks to achieve, however, and the time frame chosen could be related to the woman's planned return to work.

Nursing intervention and the delivery of care

Nurses working with this model will need to be guided by three things when planning interventions. First, they must be guided by the principles for intervention outlined in the RAM itself. Detailed nursing activity will, however, need to be planned using up-to-date evidence on how nurses should act in specified health care situations. Also, any intervention can only take place with the patient's consent, except in emergency situations, usually related to the physiological mode.

In principle, the RAM advocates interventions around the focal stimulus or stimuli, although other stimuli may be managed in order to promote adaptation. As stated earlier in this chapter, management of the stimuli involves altering, increasing, decreasing, removing or maintaining them so that coping is improved.

Whatever stimulus is selected for intervention, Roy and Andrews (1991) cite earlier work by McDonald and Harms (1966) as a means of emphasising the need for nurses to consider alternative modes of intervention and to make a judgement about their probable effectiveness. In other words, there is no one way to intervene, and nurses must use the available evidence to predict the likelihood of a particular consequence occurring. Efforts must always be made to minimise undesirable consequences, and the nurse's chosen strategy should meet with the approval of the patient.

The nurse working in the young people's sexual health clinic has ascertained that the focal stimulus prompting the young man to seek advice is the recent news that a friend is HIV positive. In order to maintain his adaptive behaviour of seeking appropriate advice, the nurse may carry out checks to ensure that the clinic environment appears welcoming and non-confrontational to him. She may previously have referred to the DoH's (1993) *Key Area Handbook HIV/AIDS and Sexual Health* for guidance and perhaps contacted other specialist clinics to find out what strategies are successful in encouraging attendance. She may now discuss the man's own views about the atmosphere and image engendered at the clinic to assess the chances of his attending again and to evaluate the clinic's probable appeal to other young gay men.

She will need to provide information for the man about HIV transmission and methods of reducing risk. It is likely that a range of information media, including written information and video presentations, will be available in an established clinic. The challenge for the nurse will be periodically to select the appropriate one(s) as the young man's knowledge develops. Providing information and checking that understanding has taken place will often involve more than one method of communication.

In the second example, if the woman were not to have chemotherapy, her fears about her appearance and her job security would not exist. However, refusing treatment for malignant disease is not a decision to be taken lightly, and most patients agree to treatment to avoid other serious, undesirable consequences. The nurse will therefore want to draw on current knowledge about the side-effects of the planned treatment and their expected duration. The ward area may have suitable texts such as *Body Image: Nursing Concepts and Care* (Price, 1990), as well as recent research articles.

To address the focal stimulus of the fear of a change of body image in the short term, the nurse may need to intervene to minimise the hair loss and help the patient make choices about the best way to cope with the alopecia expected to occur. Depending on the woman's level of fear and anxiety, the nurse may act as an advocate to encourage her to discuss drug options with the oncologist. Some chemotherapeutic agents produce more hair loss than others, and Price (1990) outlines some of the alternatives to baldness, including scarves and wigs.

In the longer term, the nurse may make sure that opportunities exist for a discussion of the woman's job and her perception of the probable impact of her looking different. The nurse may need to enlist the help of an experienced counsellor to talk through the issues of concern. In this instance, it is the residual stimulus being addressed, and as such, considerable time and support may be required as people are usually reluctant to change their more enduring beliefs.

Evaluation

Evaluation is intimately associated with the planning stage of the nursing process as it involves revisiting the goals set and seeing whether they have been achieved. There are also links to the assessment stage as the skills needed, for example interviewing and direct observation, are the same. During evaluation, the nurse will maintain a keen interest in the patient's adaptation level to see whether behaviour has remained or become more effective.

By providing information, the nurse will hope, in the short term, to increase the young man's knowledge and understanding about HIV and its transmission and thereby decrease his anxiety. Goal achievement may centre on his ability to explain to the nurse what HIV is, its modes of transmission and the precautions that can protect people, especially those related to safer sex with a male partner. Self-reported feelings about his anxiety level may be the best guide for the nurse to know whether he is worrying less about his and his partner's safety.

In the longer term, the nurse may evaluate goal achievement by keeping a record of the man's attendance at the clinic and ultimately by his decision that he no longer requires contact with the nurse to cope effectively with his concerns about HIV transmission.

As is often the case when trying to help people adapt to changes in, or perceived threats to, their lifestyle, increasing their knowledge of what is happening can be a useful strategy. For the woman with malignant disease, the nurse will evaluate the goal related to knowledge by asking the woman to explain her treatment options and their probable effect. A goal of knowledge can often be evaluated by encouraging the person to explain to someone else what is happening. This will sometimes be a close friend or relative. In relation to the self-concept mode in the RAM, the woman's confidence in herself and in her sense of control may be significantly improved if she can explain to her husband, for example, what is planned.

The nurse may also directly observe the woman's sleep pattern, perhaps also using a sleep chart with the patient. She may measure the woman's blood pressure periodically to assess whether it has lowered with decreased anxiety, and she may question her about her own assessment of her anxiety level. Her fear of the planned treatment is unlikely to be removed, but it may be altered to become more manageable or reduced to an acceptable level.

The longer-term goal related to the woman's job fears may also rely in part on her perceived feelings, but may ultimately be evaluated by her willingness to resume her career with confidence.

It is not always the case that goal achievement is found at evaluation. If a goal is not achieved, the nurse will need to discover why. Possible problems identified by Roy and Andrews (1991) include incomplete or inaccurate assessment data, the setting of unrealistic goals and inappropriate intervention strategies.

For the RAM to be credible to practising nurses, it needs thoughtful and rigorous evaluation over time. Such summative evaluation will be enhanced if the RAM is used in a variety of care settings and with different kinds of people, both patients and nurses. Nurses who aim to evaluate the model's utility will also need to talk to people, perhaps patients, relatives and colleagues, about the appropriateness of the concept of adaptation that underpins the RAM. Is this idea useful, for example, in helping to understand and provide care for people across different health care situations?

References

Andrews, H.A. and Roy, C. (1991) 'The nursing process according to the Roy adaptation model.' In Roy and Andrews (1991) *The Roy Adaption Model: The Definitive Statement*. Norwalk, CT, Appleton & Lange.

Bertalanffy, L. von (1968) *General Systems Theory*. New York, Brazillier.

Department of Health (1993) *Key Area Handbook HIV/AIDS and Sexual Health*. Heywood, Lancashire, DoH.

Helson, H. (1964) *Adaptation Level Theory*. New York, Harper & Row.

Lutjens, L.R.J. (1995) Callista Roy: an adaptation model framework. In McQuiston, C.M. and Webb, A.A. (eds) *Foundations of Nursing Theory: Contributions of 12 Key Theorists*. California, Sage.

McDonald, F. and Harms, M. (1966) Theoretical model for an experimental curriculum. *Nursing Outlook*, **14**(8): 48–51.

Price, B. (1990) *Body Image: Nursing Concepts and Care*. London, Prentice Hall.

Rambo, B.J. (1984) *Adaptation Nursing: Assessment and Intervention*. Philadelphia, W.B. Saunders.

Roy, C. (1976) *Introduction to Nursing: An Adaptation Model*. Englewood Cliffs, NJ, Prentice-Hall.

Roy, C. and Andrews, H.A. (1991) *The Roy Adaptation Model: The Definitive Statement*. Norwalk, CT, Appleton & Lange.

Roy, C. and McLeod, D. (1981) Theory of person as an adaptive system. In Roy, C. and Roberts, S.L. (eds) *Theory Construction in Nursing: An Adaptation Model*. Englewood Cliffs, NJ, Prentice-Hall.

Roy, C. and Roberts, S. (1981) *Theory Construction in Nursing: An Adaptation Model*. Englewood Cliffs, NJ, Prentice-Hall.

Chapter 8 Orem's self-care model of nursing

Unlike the models of nursing we have looked at so far, that developed by Dorothea Orem emphasises not the subsystems within people but the person as a whole and his or her unique capacity to undertake self-care. For Orem (1995), self-care links to the capabilities that adults have to regulate their own functioning and development. The power to engage in self-care is called self-care agency. In ill-health, an imbalance between the power to produce self-care and the demand for care can lead to what Orem calls a 'self-care deficit'. Nursing has a key role to play in remedying this kind of deficit. In her later writing, Orem also identified what she calls dependent-care, namely the power and capability to care for others. A gap between the power to satisfy dependent-care and the demand for this kind of care in others is what is called a 'dependent-care deficit'. Nursing also has an important role to play in satisfying this kind of deficit.

Dorothea Orem practised as a nurse for many years before becoming Director of the school of nursing at Providence Hospital, Detroit in 1940. Between 1949 and 1960, she worked for the Indiana State Board of Health and for the US Department of Health, Education and Welfare in Washington. She later taught at the Catholic University of America, and after leaving there, established her own consultancy firm in 1970. Her first book, entitled *Nursing: Concepts of Practice,* was published in 1971, and a fifth edition of this same text was published in 1995, some 11 years after her retirement. Today, Orem continues to work on the conceptual development of her self-care deficit nursing theory, as it is now known.

Key components of care

The nature of people

According to Orem, humans are knowers and thinkers, ever ready to appraise the situations in which they find themselves and act accordingly. They are capable of self-determined actions and can deliberate on a course of action even when they feel emotionally pulled in an opposite direction. Above all, they are unitary beings who act deliberatively in the pursuit of goals. Many of these ideas, which were first identified by Orem in the early 1970s, draw on the work of Arnold (1960) who was interested in the nature of what he termed 'deliberate action' and the relationship between personality and emotion.

Orem also suggests that people have the potential to acquire knowledge and skills for, and to maintain the motivation necessary to undertake, self-care and the care of dependent family members. Self-care is what maintains an equilibrium between the fulfilment of what Orem calls 'universal self-care needs' and the self-care abilities that an individual possesses to meet these. Eight universal self-care requisites or needs are highlighted by Orem's model (Figure 8.1). There is no fixed way of meeting these needs, and individuals vary greatly in the way in which they aim to satisfy them.

1. Sufficient intake of air
2. Sufficient intake of water
3. Sufficient intake of food
4. Satisfactory eliminative functions
5. Activity balanced with rest
6. Balance between solitude and social interaction
7. Prevention of hazards to human life, human functioning and human well-being
8. Promotion of human functioning and development within social groups in accordance with human potential, known human limitations and the desire for 'normalcy'

Figure 8.1   Orem's universal self-care needs

A person's ability to undertake self-care is influenced by a range of factors, including age, gender, developmental state, sociocultural orientation, family factors, patterns of living, environmental factors and the availability and adequacy of resources for self-care (Orem, 1991). Crucially, however, injury, illness and disease may create additional demands for self-care, and this is where nursing has a particular role to play.

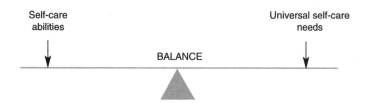

Figure 8.2   A healthy individual

A healthy person is likely to have sufficient self-care abilities to meet their universal self-care needs. Such a situation can be represented diagrammatically as in Figure 8.2. However, an individual who is ill will have additional demands for self-care. Orem calls these demands 'health deviation self-care needs'. Three types of health deviation self-care need are of particular importance:

1. Those relating to changes in a person's physical structure
2. Those linked to changes in physical function
3. Those connected to changes in behaviour.

A change in physical structure might be associated with a skin laceration or an eye infection. A change in physical function might accompany a limb fracture or might occur when a woman in middle age experiences the menopause. Behavioural changes could include a reduction in physical activity or an increase in the number of cigarettes smoked daily. Provided that a person can meet any additional demands created by health deviation self-care needs from existing self-care abilities, the overall balance is likely to be maintained and nursing will not be required. When she or he cannot do this, nursing intervention is needed (Figure 8.3).

A further set of health care needs, what Orem describes as 'developmental self-care needs', are those linked to particular stages of growth and development. They might include the needs of a pregnant woman or the ability of a child to understand what a nurse is saying about his care. When these, together with universal self-care needs, outweigh the individual's store of self-care abilities, nursing intervention may also be needed (Figure 8.4).

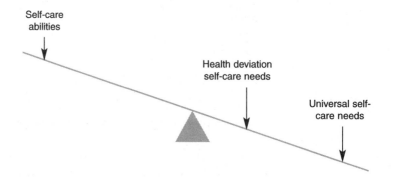

Figure 8.3   An individual in need of nursing intervention

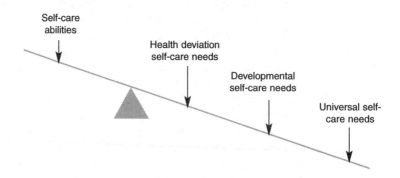

Figure 8.4   An individual in need of nursing intervention

What Orem calls 'therapeutic self-care demand' is the sum total of the universal self-care needs, the developmental self-care needs and the health deviation self-care needs that an individual possesses. Therapeutic self-care demand is normally met through the self-care agency of the individual, and the dependent-care agency provided to that individual by other adults (usually family members) and the intervention provided by the nurse.

The causes of problems likely to require nursing intervention

Nursing intervention is indicated when individuals (or their relatives and significant others) are unable to achieve or maintain a balance between their self-care abilities and the demands that are made on these. When demands for self-care exceed self-care abilities, nursing is required. Nursing interventions aim to restore the balance between self-care abilities and the demands that are made on them (Figure 8.5).

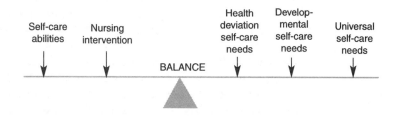

Figure 8.5 An individual in receipt of nursing intervention

It is important to recognise that a deficit between an individual's self-care abilities and the demands placed on him or her is not in itself a disorder (Cavanagh, 1991), although it may give rise to problems of structure, function and behaviour that call for nursing care to be instigated.

The nature of assessment – nursing history

Orem rarely uses the term 'assessment' in her writing. Instead she favours nurses preparing what she describes as a 'nursing history'. However, her commitment to the use of the nursing process as a means of planning and delivering care means that we can regard this activity as being synonymous with what is elsewhere described as assessment. Taking a nursing history aims to identify whether or not a self-care deficit is present. It involves comparing present demands for self-care with the abilities that individuals have to provide it.

The nurse needs to calculate present and future therapeutic self-care demand by focusing on each universal, developmental and health deviation self-care requisite in turn. She then needs to determine the person's self-care and dependent-care agency. Finally, she needs to calculate whether or not there is a self-care or dependent-care deficit, including its magnitude and the primary reasons for it. A number of issues may need to be further assessed in connection with identifying such causes. These include identifying whether an individual possesses the *knowledge* necessary to respond to self-care demands and assessing his or her *motivation, development* and *past experience*.

It is also necessary to identify whether the individual's present state allows for a safe involvement in self-care. This may not always be true, as in the case of someone with short-term memory loss who retains the physical ability to feed himself but may forget to check on the temperature of the food presented. Assessment should be neither haphazard nor intuitive; indeed, in this respect, Orem draws specific attention to what she terms the 'technologic-professional role' of the nurse. Assessment is, however, a continuing process, more information being gathered as the relationship between nurse and patient develops. Given the stress that this model places on dependent-care as well as self-care, family members and significant others have an important role to play throughout assessment.

The nature of planning and goal-setting – planning care

Following the taking of a nursing history, nurse and patient embark upon a process of 'planning'. Orem calls this the point at which *prescriptive operations* are made. These specify the care measures that will be used in order to meet therapeutic self-care demand, and the means that will be used to meet particular self-care needs. The relative contribution of nurse and patient to meeting these needs is also decided upon.

A significant part of the planning involves negotiating with the patient whether nursing intervention is to be *wholly compensatory, partly compensatory* or *supportive-educative*. Orem calls this process 'nursing system design'. Thus, in preparing a patient to undertake self-care, the nurse can act for the patient completely, can share certain tasks with the patient or can intervene in a way that is broadly consultative and facilitative.

Planning and goal-setting involves giving careful considera-tion to the timing of proposed interventions and the place in which they will occur. The appropriateness of the nursing envi-ronment will often have to be considered, along with the avail-ability of appropriate equipment and staff.

The focus of nursing intervention during implementation of the care plan

Implementing the care plan is likely to involve both nurse and patient undertaking activities to help meet therapeutic self-care demand as well as particular self-care needs. The patient's family and significant others are often involved in this process. At least six broad ways can be envisaged in which nurses can assist in implementing a care plan (Figure 8.6), each of which requires a complementary role from the patient. It is important to recognise that Orem's model assumes that patients are willing and able to adopt certain roles and that they desire to achieve self-care.

---

1. Doing for or acting for another
2. Guiding or directing another
3. Providing physical support
4. Providing psychological support
5. Providing an environment supportive of development
6. Teaching another

Figure 8.6   Six methods of helping

The nature of evaluation

The main criterion to be used in evaluating the success of care is whether a patient's or family's ability to perform self-care improves. To measure this, a careful check may need to be made of each goal to ascertain the degree to which it is being met. In general terms, a move from nursing intervention that is wholly compensatory to that which seeks to support patients in the performance of self-care should be taken as a sign of success.

A patient's success in maintaining a balance between self-care demands and self-care abilities depends both on an increased capacity to perform self-care activities and on changes in self-care demands. Orem calls this latter kind of change 'recovery' – a term she uses in a way broadly similar to its more general use within the medical model of care.

The role of the nurse

Orem's model of nursing sees nurses first and foremost as 'helpers', people who help others do for themselves or help family members to learn how to help those with care limitations. They help those in need of care to overcome health-derived limitations. While their actions may occasionally be wholly compensatory, they more usually aim to complement the individual's need and ability to undertake self-care. Nurses intervene in patients' lives to help individuals to sustain health, recover from injury or disease and cope with the effects of illness.

Using Orem's model

The emphasis on self-care in Orem's model of nursing demands a particular nurse–patient relationship. The word 'care' could be taken to mean that the individual (or self) has a key role only in the intervention stage of the nursing process. In other words, planned care is given by the individual him or herself. Such an interpretation would be an injustice to Orem's model, which, as has been identified above, is committed to self-care throughout the process of nursing and also acknowledges the importance of dependent-care agency. It is these two elements, self-care *through-out* the process of nursing and *dependent*-care agency, that mean that the nurse–patient relationship in Orem's model is rather different from that in the other models so far considered.

To illustrate these two important features, we will look first at how the model might be used with a woman admitted for gynaecological surgery, focusing only on her particular concern about pain relief. Second, we will look at how the model might contribute to the care of a preschool age child admitted for day surgery for the removal of his tonsils. The first example will focus on the involvement of the self (patient/client) throughout an episode of care, as Orem's model recommends. The second will include some of the issues raised when adults care for those who are dependent on them.

Nursing history

Although Orem tends to use the term 'nursing history' (Orem, 1995), what she describes is very similar to the more commonly used term, 'assessment'. Orem identifies two main sections to the nursing history. The first section considers both the particular self-care situation of the patient, including any changes in the therapeutic self-care demand, and the patient's personal focus of self-care. Section 2 was developed by Orem in cooperation with Evelyn Vardiman (Orem, 1995: 422) and looks at more general activities and patterns of living. This section emerged from a particular need for information to assist day centre clients with chronic mental illness. Orem acknowledges that nurses using a nursing history with sensitivity will be able to select what is needed in a specific situation. Sometimes one section will be more relevant than the other. Sometimes only parts of each section will be needed.

More than some other nurse theorists, Orem recognises that nurses have decisions to make throughout the care process. She does not see them as constrained by her model but more as knowledgeable practitioners who should be capable of implementing the model sensitively and creatively as each situation demands. Orem acknowledges that nurses should not gather large amounts of irrelevant data but should tailor the taking of a nursing history to the needs of the individual patient. She also recognises that there are differences between those nurses with experience and others. It may thus be the case that newly qualified nurses, or nurses new to working with a particular model, or nurses new to a clinical speciality, may take longer to gather information and may gather more data than an experienced nurse might find necessary.

Nursing Models and Nursing Practice

Nursing history – section 1

The nurse will initially be interested in changes in the therapeutic self-care demand and in the individual nature of the person's self-care agency. Areas to be explored will therefore include any alterations to self-care that the person has made in the light of present health circumstances. Such alterations might include curtailing or limiting certain activities, or taking medications. The nurse should also encourage the person to identify any special contribution to meeting the therapeutic care demand that nurses can make. To gather information about the individual's self-care agency, questions to adults should focus on the development of self-care abilities over time and on any present help being received. In addition, the nurse will ask about past episodes of illness or disability and how these were managed.

In the first example, a woman has been admitted for elective gynaecological surgery. In relation to the therapeutic self-care demand, the nurse might discover that, because of heavy periods, the woman has been taking an oral iron preparation and has felt very tired. She might therefore have given up certain physical activities such as walking and swimming and taken additional rest during the day. At this stage, the nurse will also ascertain what the woman believes her problem is and what operative procedure she expects to be carried out.

Orem advocates that nursing documentation should include patients' statements about themselves. This serves to reinforce the importance of self, in this case demonstrated by the person's own understanding and choice of words. To record verbatim what someone understands about their present health situation can often be helpful to subsequent care and is in keeping with UKCC advice that records should be written in terms that patients can understand (UKCC, 1998). Such records detail the words that the patient is likely to use when talking about the planned treatment, and also serve to identify any lack of knowledge or misunderstanding at an early stage. It is during this part of the nursing history that the nurse may also ascertain how able the woman feels to talk to medical staff about her current condition and treatment and their impact on her self-care abilities.

When asked about any special contribution that the woman believes the nurse can make during this planned episode of care, she may particularly focus on postoperative pain and her concern about how it will be managed. She may have had previous unrelated surgery and have experienced the distress caused by poor pain relief. This will alert the nurse to the need for detailed information about this past episode so that care can be more appropriate on this occasion.

The focus on self-care can be maintained by asking the woman what contribution she feels able to make to her current care and identifying any aspects that she thinks may prove difficult or stressful. Here, Orem's model recognises that meeting the therapeutic self-care demand involves more than just completing a set of tasks. It is also concerned with how a person feels about the activities and, importantly from a nursing point of view, how able someone feels both to cooperate when help is being offered and to guide the carer.

In the second example, the nursing history will focus on the needs of the child who is to have his tonsils removed and on the needs of his parents. History-taking will include gathering data on the parents' ability to care safely and confidently for their son on discharge. It is primarily the parents' needs to ensure a safe discharge home that will be the focus here in order to illustrate dependent-care agency and the nursing role that complements it.

At this stage, the nurse will also ask the parents about any recent changes in their son's therapeutic self-care demand and how they have coped with these. She may discover that the little boy becomes very distressed when his throat is sore, and that when this happens, he is very reluctant to drink. She will want to know if the parents have managed all the care during such episodes or whether they have received help from nurses in the community or from other health care workers or family members. This will provide important information about the parents' abilities to act as dependent-care agents at times when their son is not as self-caring as usual. The nurse may also ask about any other children in an effort to assess the overall care demand that might be present in the home. In this example, however, the main focus of the nursing history will be on the second section.

Nursing history – section 2

According to Orem (1995), section 2 of the nursing history considers conditions and patterns of living by eliciting information about, for example, where and with whom the person lives, how time is spent each day and the routine meeting of the eight universal self-care requisites. Judgements need to be made about the degree of detail required in each area. Living accommodation and environmental factors will sometimes be very significant to care but at other times be less so. During this part of the nursing history, the nurse will also decide the degree of detail needed on how the eight universal self-care needs are met. She may ask some questions about each one and, on the basis of this information, discuss with the person whether more detail is required. A generally healthy, and therefore self-caring, adult admitted for elective surgery may not need the same amount of detail recorded for each requisite as someone who is critically ill.

In the example of the woman approaching surgery for heavy periods, the nurse may establish that the woman has no concerns about her home circumstances, and a brief description will suffice to confirm that discharge home will pose no particular threat to the woman's postoperative recovery. She may also find that the woman has never smoked and has no breathing problems (universal self-care requisite 1) and eats and drinks a full range of foods and fluids (universal self-care requisites 2 and 3). It is, therefore, not necessary to seek detailed information about, for example, her ability to prepare meals or the exact amount and type of food eaten at each meal. However, she may have experienced a problem with the fourth universal self-care requisite (related to elimination) associated both with menstruation and with taking oral iron, which can cause constipation or diarrhoea (Govoni and Hayes, 1990). In this instance, more information will be helpful about any successful strategies that she is currently adopting and any measures that she has not found helpful. It may be that other information (for example particular foodstuffs taken) will be recorded here, in relation to elimination rather than to food intake.

The woman has already identified changes in her levels of activity and rest (universal self-care requisite 5), and these changes may also have affected her social activities and contacts (universal self-care requisite 6). A problem has been anticipated in relation to universal self-care requisite 7, namely that postoperative pain could be a hazard to her well-being. The precise recording of pain at the assessment or nursing history stage is regarded as problematic by some nurses. Most models do not specifically address the place of pain when using a model in practice. No model cites pain as a central feature of the nature of people, although the difficulty of assessing pain, and intervening to manage it, is a preoccupation with many health professionals. As a general rule, pain is best considered in Orem's model in association with the self-care requisite(s) it most affects.

Orem uses the word 'normalcy' in relation to requisite 8. It is unfortunate that the word is not included in the glossary of Orem's most recent text as it poses some problems of definition. However, elsewhere in the text she defines it thus:

Normalcy is used in the sense of that which is essentially human and that which is in accord with the genetic and constitutional characteristics and talents of individuals. (Orem, 1995: 192)

For the woman approaching surgery, the nurse may ask her how she feels about the changes that will occur to her body structure and whether she perceives any threat to her self-concept. Women appear to vary considerably in how concerned they are about internal, non-visible changes, for example following hysterectomy (Dickson and Henriques, 1994), and hospital nurses now have less experience of the effects on patients with the decreasing lengths of inpatient stay.

In the second example, the nurse will focus particularly on section 2 of the nursing history because information about living conditions and the routines of the parents' self-care agency will be crucial. She will need to know some information about the accommodation in which the family live, but by focusing questions on what the parents foresee as the self-care demand following discharge, an experienced nurse should not need to gather large amounts of irrelevant data. For example, by asking the parents to describe the preparations they have made for the first postoperative night, the nurse should obtain useful data that show where the areas of concern might be. Thus, if the parents outline adequate plans to ensure that one of them can sleep in the boy's room, the nurse does not need to record more detail about bedroom space.

Information will be sought about any potential hazards in the home environment. In this particular example, the nurse will want to know whether anyone in the household smokes, the availability of suitable drinks and food for a child following tonsil removal, and the current health status of others living in the house. She will ask what arrangements have been made for meeting the dependent care needs of the child and will check how many adults will be sleeping in the home during the first postoperative night.

It is not likely that detailed information will be gathered about the usual meeting of all the child's self-care needs as the parents are the normal agents and will be able to identify any particular concerns. However, the nurse may ask about the child's sleeping behaviour and about the kind of activities that usually entertain him. It may become apparent that the little boy dislikes going to bed at night until he is very sleepy and that the parents are worried that he should perhaps go to bed as soon as he is discharged from hospital.

Planning care

Orem (1995) does not offer much detail in her writing about the nature of planning when using her model. However, a continued commitment on the part of the nurse to the importance of self-care throughout the nursing process should ensure that this stage can be successfully tailored to the patient's needs. Cavanagh (1991) has advocated the use of a common document on which to formulate a plan, while at the same time arguing for variety and flexibility in care planning. The potential for flexibility in using Orem's model hinges on the patient's unique contribution to this stage in the care process and on the value that Orem places on nurses as knowledgeable practitioners able to make care decisions.

Thus, the planning stage provides another opportunity for the model's commitment to self-care to be demonstrated. Orem advocates that, whenever possible, plans to meet self-care needs should be discussed and agreed with the patient. She describes the nurse–patient relationship as being *contractual* in nature (Orem 1995). Careful inclusion of the patient in such discussions helps to value the individuality (self) of the person and to plan appropriate care actions. Plans should include information about the amount, and in some cases the precise timing, of the required nurse–patient contact and the relative contributions that will be made by the patient, the nurse and any others involved in care. Timing will be more important to some patients than to others. When nursing care is being given in the patient's home, there may be personal and environmental commitments and constraints that the nurse will need to take into account when planning visits. In a hospital setting, it is often important to liaise with other health professionals as well as the patient to ensure that activities do not clash during the day.

For the woman approaching surgery, the nursing history highlighted a concern about postoperative pain relief. A nurse familiar with pain-relieving measures, and the resources available within her clinical area, can discuss the various options with the woman. The planning stage will be particularly crucial for this woman's care as her confidence that effective pain relief will be achieved in the postoperative period is likely to colour all aspects of her preoperative preparation. Together, the patient and nurse may conclude that the provision of patient-controlled analgesia (PCA) will best meet the woman's needs, especially if the nursing history shows that she wishes to be involved as much as possible with all elements of her care. As a result of these discussions, the nurse will need to liaise with the anaesthetist to confirm that PCA can be set up. Once this has been ascertained, she can plan ways in which to familiarise the woman with the equipment that will be used in the postoperative period and to ensure that she understands the procedure.

For the child to be discharged safely following surgery, the nurse will discuss plans to address concerns raised by the parents during the taking of the nursing history and will agree plans to ensure that they have as much guidance as possible about postoperative care. The focus here cannot be entirely based on concerns discovered at assessment as the parents may have a knowledge deficit in relation to what might occur after surgery and the actions they might need to take.

The nurse has already discovered that, when his throat is sore, the child has previously been reluctant to drink. Also, his parents have expressed the opinion that he should go to bed when he returns home but know that in normal circumstances he would be unlikely to want this. When talking with the parents, the nurse will therefore plan with them what measures might encourage their son to drink. Discussion will probably focus on the adequacy of pain relief, the provision of drinks most favoured by the child and any special cups or mugs that might influence his willingness to drink. As part of the plan to meet his need for fluids, the nurse may reassure the parents that their son will only be discharged when they and the nurse think that pain relief is good enough. This might be shown by the little boy drinking small amounts willingly and without distress.

Plans may also be discussed that take note of the fact that the little boy dislikes going to bed and that it is the parents' view that he will need to be in bed following discharge. The nurse may suggest that safe alternatives to going to his own bed should be considered in light of the circumstances at home, for example a sofa in the family living room, or the parents' bed.

Orem cites the need for dependent-care agents to develop capabilities to recognise emergency situations and to act promptly and effectively (Orem 1995). The nurse will decide with the parents the most appropriate times for such concerns with regard to their son's care to be talked about. According to Orem, as the period of care progresses, dependent-care agency is developed to meet the emerging needs of the child. Therefore the parents may be more ready to discuss care following discharge once surgery has taken place. The nurse, however, might suggest some activities for the preoperative period so that there is time for the information to be considered and revisited.

Casey (1994), among others, sees child care as being best carried out by families whenever possible. The considerable ability that families and others sometimes develop to care for a dependant is sometimes given as a reason to challenge the need for all nurses to be trained over an extended period. Qualified nurses can care for all kinds of people with a variety of health-related problems. In addition, they can assess the likelihood of problems or complications arising and act accordingly. Thus, while a family member or friend might become the most skilled helper of a particular person, the skills are not readily or safely transferable to anyone else. Such an excellent contribution to one individual's care is therefore not a convincing argument for the increased use of non-qualified personnel in nursing roles.

Nursing intervention and the delivery of care

Orem regards nursing intervention as being complementary to that which the patient or dependent-care agent can achieve. In other words, nurses act in a variety of ways to make up for any deficiencies or deficits in capabilities. This can range from wholly compensatory through partially compensatory to supportive-educative care.

As with all models of nursing, information about precisely how to intervene cannot be found and should not be sought in

Orem's model itself. Models do not provide information about the detailed ways in which nurses can intervene. Instead, guidance is provided about the types of activity in which nurses might engage as they seek to assist someone to meet his or her self-care demands.

For the woman concerned about postoperative pain relief, the main focus of nursing intervention in relation to this in the preoperative period will be to familiarise her with the PCA equipment, particularly with the hand-held control that she will use to obtain analgesia. The nurse will therefore ensure that there is a hand control for the woman to handle and she will be present to demonstrate the action required, to answer any questions and to provide encouragement and support. If it is available, she may provide literature for the woman and her family on the use of PCA, as well as showing her and talking with her about the measuring tool to be used to assess her postoperative pain and evaluate its relief.

In this way, a number of Orem's helping methods will be in evidence. For example, the nurse will be using different teaching abilities to demonstrate a skill and to promote understanding. She will also be providing psychological support, ideally in an environment that the woman finds conducive to learning.

In the immediate postoperative period, the nurse may need to act for the woman if she requests pain relief but is still too sleepy from the anaesthetic to activate the control herself. This is likely to be for a very brief period, and the early re-establishment of self-care with regard to the administration of analgesia should be facilitated by high-quality preoperative preparation.

In the second example, the parents will remain the dependent-care agents during their son's inpatient stay and will care for him alongside nursing staff. This provides an ongoing opportunity for the nurse to add information to the nursing history and carry out the agreed plan. Prior to surgery, she may provide a discharge information sheet specifically designed for dependent-care agents taking a child home after tonsillectomy carried out in a day care unit. If this has been given before admission, she may check that the parents still have the information. Such standard advice sheets provide a useful focus of discussion on safe post-discharge care but need to be supplemented with additional information pertinent to the particular needs of the child and the concerns of his parents.

Much of the nursing intervention in this example will be fulfilled through the helping methods of guiding and directing, providing psychological support and teaching. Once the little boy has returned from the operating theatre, the nurse will guide and direct the parents as necessary as they care for their son. In particular, the nurse will be concerned to ensure that the parents are confident in those aspects of their son's care that will continue at home. Thus, if, for example, a short-term intravenous infusion is in progress, the nurse might act for the parents in any activities associated with this in the knowledge that it will be discontinued before discharge.

However, it will be important for the parents to be actively involved in care associated with pain relief, hydration and nutrition, and observing for any complications. The nurse should provide psychological support by being present or readily available as the postoperative period progresses and by asking the parents how confident they feel about caring for their son. When a particular need arises for intervention, she should discuss what can be done with the parents so that they become familiar with the options available and confident in how to select those which are most appropriate.

It is often helpful to rehearse verbally with the parents the probable sequence of events on discharge home so that they are as well prepared as possible. In this example, the nurse may discuss alternatives to bed as an environment of safety until the boy agrees that he is sleepy. She may need to reassure the parents that going to bed is not beneficial in itself and that if their son is content, for example, on a sofa with other family members around, that is an acceptable alternative. A child will sometimes take an interest in such dialogue, and he should be given honest answers to questions asked, in a way that he can understand. Some children may benefit from discharge advice sheets developed specifically for them using pictures and words appropriate to their stage of development.

By the time the little boy is considered well enough to go home, his parents should be caring for him completely and should be able to explain to the nurse the main emphasis of his care over the subsequent few days. They should be able to say in what circumstances they would seek medical or nursing assistance and how they would access an appropriate source of help. Whenever possible, they should have access by telephone to the nurse who looked after their son or to an informed colleague, but staff on a day care unit are often not available at night.

Evaluation

Orem does not write specifically about evaluation but repeatedly mentions the need for self-care demands to be met. Therefore, evaluation will focus on the degree to which deficits in the patient's self-care abilities have been satisfied and will also consider whether or not the method of achievement is or has been acceptable to the patient. This further serves to maintain attention on the importance of self in the total care process. Evaluation may be concerned with identifying the relative contributions to meeting the self-care demand made by nurses, the patient and the patient's family. For self-care to be re-established, there will need to be an increasing contribution from the patient or a capable other, with a corresponding decrease in nursing intervention. Orem (1995) recommends the recording of progress notes, which should include nurses' judgements about the patient's progress towards meeting the self-care demand. Inclusion, whenever possible, of the patient's own judgement is crucial to maintaining the importance of self.

The adequacy of pain control will form a major part of evaluation for the woman who has had gynaecological surgery. Information documented in relation to the measuring tool for pain experienced will serve as a regular reassessment or evaluation throughout the postoperative period. The frequency with which this is recorded will vary; it may be, for example, half-hourly in the early postoperative period. Other indicators of the adequacy of pain control may be included in the progress notes, for example the ease with which the patient moves and carries out breathing and leg exercises.

In the longer term, the nurse will want to know more about how the whole experience of managing the postoperative pain was evaluated by the patient. This will include the adequacy of the preoperative preparation, particularly with regard to PCA. She may ask the patient to comment on the appropriateness of this method of pain relief. Information such as this maintains the important focus on the central concept of self-care. Although a relatively simple tool can be used to evaluate the adequacy of pain relief, a nurse sensitive to the philosophy of Orem's model will want to look beyond pain relief alone and consider its management within the context of self-care.

Evaluation of the care provided for the boy and his parents will also have two main components. First, the nurse will want to evaluate the success of interventions that were designed to prepare the parents to take their son home on the same day as the tonsillectomy was carried out and for them to be confident in their abilities to act as his dependent-care agents. This can be judged by observing the parents caring for the boy postoperatively and by asking them to explicate the care required on discharge. They can also be asked how confident they feel about taking him home.

Second, the nurse will want some feedback on how the parents managed at home and the progress made by their son after discharge. As further contact in person may not be usual, the nurse might construct a short questionnaire for the parents to take home and complete on a specified postoperative day.

Working with Orem's model raises questions about creative ways of developing the notion of self-care in health care settings. The more that adults are involved in all aspects of the nursing process, the more nurses may be motivated to develop innovative ways of fostering the promotion of self. For example, patient involvement could be extended to include some patients completing much of their own assessment documentation. If this were to be the case, self-assessment forms would need to be constructed. It would not be appropriate for patients to be asked to complete nursing history documentation, which is prepared in the knowledge that a nurse is involved throughout. Self-assessment could be an innovative development in some clinical areas and might produce very reliable data. Patients being admitted electively to hospital would be able to complete a self-assessment form at home prior to coming in and without the anxiety frequently attendant on being admitted.

The emphasis within Orem's model on self, and self-care in particular, should be the focus of a summative evaluation. Early discharge from hospital and the increase of care in the community mean that a model with a clear focus on the role of self and on dependent-care agency has certain attractions. Nurses with experience of the model in a number of settings and with a variety of patients may find that the concept of self-care has much potential. Its usefulness will need to be assessed against other models with a similar emphasis, especially those that value independence. Nurses may also want to find out how much value individual patients place on the importance of self.

Summative evaluation should also consider the role of the nurse as envisaged by Orem. She sees the nursing role as complementary to that of the patient and describes nurses working alongside doctors but with different *special interests* (Orem 1995). Nurses will need to consider how appropriate this is within current health care practice in the UK and elsewhere in Europe.

References

Arnold, M.B. (1960) Deliberate action. In *Emotion and Personality*, vol. 11: *Neurological and Physiological Aspects*. New York, Columbia University Press.

Casey, A. (1994) A partnership with child and family. In Gott, M. and Moloney, B. (eds) *Child Health: A Reader*. Buckingham, Open University Press.

Cavanagh, S.J. (1991) *Orem's Model in Action*. London, Macmillan.

Dickson, A. and Henriques, N. (1994) *Hysterectomy: The Woman's View*. London, Quartet Books.

Govoni, L.E. and Hayes, J.E. (1990) *Drugs and Nursing Implications*. London, Prentice Hall.

Orem, D.E. (1991) *Nursing: Concepts of Practice*, 4th edn. St Louis, C.V. Mosby.

Orem, D.E. (1995) *Nursing: Concepts of Practice*, 5th edn. St Louis, C.V. Mosby.

United Kingdom Central Council for Nursing, Midwifery and Health Visiting (1998) *Guidelines for Records and Record Keeping*. London, UKCC.

Chapter 9 King's open systems model of nursing

Imogene King qualified as a nurse in 1945 from St John's Hospital of Nursing in St Louis, Missouri. After teaching nursing for several years, she became Assistant Director of St John's Hospital School of Nursing, St Louis before being appointed an Associate Professor of Nursing at Loyola University, Chicago. From there, she joined the Division of Nursing within the US Department of Health, Education and Welfare and then the School of Nursing at the Ohio State University, Columbus, before eventually moving to the University of South Florida in Tampa as a Professor of Nursing. Since her retirement from the University of Florida in 1990, King has continued to teach, plan care and consult on the further development of her model of nursing. Her first book, *Toward a Theory for Nursing*, was published in 1971, her second, *A Theory for Nursing: Systems, Concepts, Process*, in 1981, and her third, *Curriculum and Instruction in Nursing*, in 1986.

Debates about the relationship between theory and practice in nursing were the impetus that led King to develop her open systems model of nursing in the 1960s and 70s. In an early article, King (1964: 28) commented on what she felt was an 'anti-theoretical bias' in nursing, which had led to the development of nursing theory 'based on practical techniques – the "how" rather than the "why"'. This led her to examine more closely why nurses think and act in the way they do, and why nursing has developed in the way it has. She has done this by trying to identify the dimensions of practice that give nursing its unifying focus, codifying these and suggesting ways in which they might be applied.

Key components of care

The nature of people

According to King, the most fundamental quality shared by all human beings is their capacity to interact meaningfully with one another in the pursuit of a common goal. They can do this in many different ways: as individuals, as groups and as societies. 'Goal-related interaction', as King calls it, establishes three dynamic and interacting systems – the *personal*, the *interpersonal* and the *social*. Nurses must have good knowledge of each of these systems and their interrelationships if they are to be able to plan and deliver good-quality care.

According to King (1981: 27), the personal system is 'a unified, complex whole self who perceives, thinks, desires, imagines, decides, identifies goals and selects means to achieve them'. The personal system consists of perceptions of the self, of body image and of time and space. These perceptions influence the ways in which people present themselves and respond to others whom they meet. They also affect people's responses to situations and events. The personal system can grow and change as a person develops and matures.

The interpersonal system, on the other hand, is concerned primarily with communication and interaction. It is through communication that people can establish and work towards common goals. It is also through communication that agreement can be reached on the means of achieving agreed ends. This kind of communication, or *transaction*, is a key quality of people and their interpersonal behaviour. The interpersonal system also gives rise to roles or expected kinds of behaviour. Stress, which is a major inhibitor of growth and a threat to health, can arise from interpersonal relations and from role conflict. It can be reduced by transactions.

The social system is established by the interactions between the larger groups in which we live. Social systems are generally structured in order to ensure that activities of daily living to maintain life, health and hopefully happiness can take place within them. Communities, localities, workplaces, hospitals and other institutions are among the social systems given particular attention by King's model. Power is fundamental to social life within each of these settings and is a key factor to be taken into account when planning and delivering nursing care.

The relationship between King's three systems can be represented diagrammatically as in Figure 9.1.

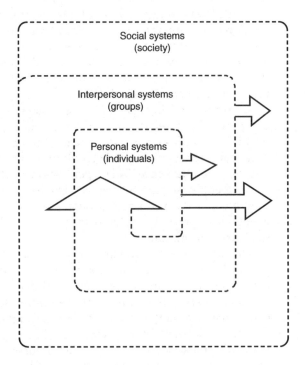

Figure 9.1   King's open systems model of nursing

The causes of problems likely to require nursing intervention

The majority of problems likely to require nursing intervention are linked to stress of one kind or another. Problems may include the inability to meet needs for daily living and the inability to function in an appropriate role. The causes of these problems may be physical, such as a temporary loss of function as a result of trauma or perhaps surgery, or more permanent changes caused by ageing and/or degenerative processes. Other causes of stress may be related to changes in personal, interpersonal and social systems. Examples might include changes in self-concept and body image, difficulties in communicating and transacting with others, and difficulties arising through a loss of empowerment. Regardless of their cause, all of these problems are likely to be associated with subjective feelings of illness or distress.

The nature of assessment – nursing history and health assessment

King's model does not distinguish as clearly as some others between assessment, planning, intervention and evaluation. Instead, she seems to favour the use of the Goal-Oriented Nursing Record, or GONR (King 1981, 1984), although she admits that most nurses work with the four-stage nursing process. Nurses working with King's model will therefore need to choose between the nursing process and the GONR. The elements of the GONR are a database, a problem list, a goal list, a plan and progress notes. For nurses using such an approach, the nursing process is thus replaced with a differently staged problem-solving process. In this chapter we will use this alternative approach since it is closer to the way of working that King herself advocates.

McKenna (1997) has argued that the nursing process is linear, but for nurses to work effectively, neither the nursing process nor the GONR should be viewed in this way. Instead, data should be periodically added to the nursing history as the nurse and patient interact. Both objective and subjective sources of information will be drawn upon. Objective data might include the results of physical examinations and laboratory tests, whereas subjective data might contain information on how a patient feels about his or her condition. The GONR has a database and a problem list in place of assessment. The database is made up of multidisciplinary information, of which the nursing part comprises the nursing history and the health assessment. Taking a nursing history and health assessment is, therefore, the first stage in the use of the model.

The nature of planning and goal setting – goal list and nursing plan

Following the taking of a nursing history and a health assessment, and in the light of the overall database and problem list, nurse and patient will together embark upon a process of 'planning'. This involves drawing up a list of goals to be achieved (the 'goal list') and a nursing plan. King (1981) sees goal attainment as part of everyday life and achievable through the human capacity to interact and to agree on the action required to fulfil a goal. She describes the performance of a variety of roles as being crucial to goal attainment. In nursing, she values mutual goal-setting by nurses and their clients/patients but acknowledges that the goals of nurses and the goals of the people for whom they care may at times not be congruent.

The focus of nursing intervention during implementation of the care plan

King sees nursing care as being reliant on both knowledge and skills of communication. For her, 'communication is the vehicle by which human relations are developed and maintained' (King, 1981: 79). She recognises the uniqueness of each individual and stresses that nursing skills need to be tailored to make them appropriate for each person. She cites many different situations in which a knowledge of communication is essential and identifies in particular the needs of children who cannot use language, the needs of elderly people and the needs of those with intractable pain.

King regards interactions that occur in a nursing context as being purposeful, with a particular emphasis on helping people to cope with a health or health-related concern. This will often involve actions associated with learning in which both the nurse and the patient become more self-aware. Such a working together holds the potential for a new kind of relationship between nurse and patient. Here, the emphasis is upon meaningful *transactions* between the patient and the nurse. Transactions involve the sharing of wants, needs and values, and require the nurse and patient to adopt appropriate roles. Successful transactions, which only occur when there is perceptual accuracy in the nurse–patient interaction, lead to a reduction of stress and anxiety, and hence contribute to patient growth and development.

The nature of evaluation – progress notes

King argues that quality care is expected by the public (King, 1981) and that there should therefore be measures of the effectiveness of care. Such effectiveness can be measured by goal attainment, and evidence for this should feature in what King calls progress notes. She sees both process and outcome as being important measures of quality assurance. King (1981) advocates the use of three different types of progress notes: narrative notes, flow sheets and final summaries or discharge notes (compare Weed, 1969).

Narrative notes detail chronologically what progress, if any, has been made towards goal attainment. Depending on the patient and the nature of the problem list and goals agreed, such notes may be prepared at several points during a 24-hour period or, might, for less acute difficulties, be recorded daily.

Flow charts are used to record routine information or for repetitive, for example hourly, recordings such as oxygen saturation levels, neurological observations or pain assessments.

Final summaries state the position with regard to each goal at the end of a period of care or when a patient is transferring to a different care environment. Within the final summary, progress with regard to each goal is documented, as is an overall summary that may also indicate any outstanding goals.

The role of the nurse

Nurses working with King's model can adopt a variety of roles. They may have a strategic role to play in relation to human growth and development, and in the planning and delivery of health care services. They have an important role to play in alleviating health-related stress and a further part to play in helping people to cope with changes in their daily activities. Above all, however, they are vital in communication and interaction as facilitators of meaningful health-related transactions.

Using King's model

King (1981) suggests that people have three fundamental health needs: the need for information, the need for preventive care and the need for care when they are unable to help themselves. The two examples we will offer in this chapter illustrate these health needs. First, we will consider the case of a child, who fears injections, being admitted to hospital for an overnight stay. Here, relevant information and action are required to prevent distress. In the second example, a man being cared for at home wants to prepare for the time when he may no longer be able to make decisions about his own care.

King acknowledges that nurses and doctors often have rather different goals in health care, and she advocates good communication and cooperation between professionals to maximise the patient benefit to be achieved through coordinated teamwork. In essence, she sees the goal of nursing as promoting health, preventing disease and caring for those who are ill, incapacitated or dying. Doctors, on the other hand, seek to diagnose, treat and cure diseases and illnesses. Both the examples cited in this chapter demonstrate the need for nurses to work in cooperation with others.

Nursing history and health assessment

King recognises that the use of her model in different care settings or with different types of person may mean that the information gathered for the database varies. Patients may sometimes be assessed primarily in terms of the medical diagnosis assigned to them, sometimes particular nursing care needs might predominate, as with an unconscious patient, and at other times the most important element of assessment may be an examination of someone's activities of daily living in order to determine the level of independence being achieved.

It is clear that the nursing history and health assessment need to be focused on the particular concerns and current needs of the person involved. King has argued that theory should guide practice, and the scope and extent of a particular patient assessment should therefore be influenced by what is required rather than by what the nurse is able to do. Nurses working with this model should therefore begin the data-gathering process by agreeing with the patient, whenever possible, what the main thrust of taking a nursing history and health assessment is to be. King also values input into data-gathering from sources other than the patient, including family and social workers.

The interaction between individuals is central to King's model and is nowhere more crucial than during the early contact of nurse and patient. Here, the interpersonal system is very important as verbal and non-verbal methods of communication are used to enable the nurse to understand the patient better, and to move them both towards agreeing goals for care.

Indeed, the centrality of understanding each other's perceptions is noted by a number of writers on King's model, including Burney (1992) and DiNardo (1989).

In the first example, a nursing history and health assessment are to be carried out for a child recently admitted to hospital for a surgical procedure necessitating an overnight stay. The child's parent(s) will be asked for their view about the child's general health state. While it is important not to miss key aspects of health data, it is also important to tailor the assessment to the child's own needs. For a short hospital admission when a parent is staying, a normally active child, whose parents state that he is healthy, does not need to have a detailed account made of every aspect of his activities of daily living. It is much more relevant for an appropriately focused history to be taken that addresses his current needs. The nurse will want to know, for example, whether he has been in hospital before and how he felt about it. Depending on the child's age and willingness to talk to the nurse, some of these data may come from the child himself; additional information can sought from his parents. King advocates recording data on previous episodes in hospital and on the experience of hospitalisation. The database form published in her 1981 text is designed for use with adult patients. For a child, the nurse will want to know about anything that particularly worried the child, anything that he especially liked or disliked and any problems following discharge home.

In this example, the parents indicate that the child has a fear of injections but they do not relate this to a previous hospitalisation. As is often the case, the cause of a specific fear may not be recognised even though it probably exists. Further questioning of the child and his parents may ascertain information of importance, in particular what behaviour occurs when the child is frightened, what particular nurse or doctor activity stimulates the fear and what, if anything, has previously helped.

For example, the nurse needs to know whether being told that an injection is required causes a problem or whether it is the procedure itself that does so. She also needs to know whether the child fears being hurt. Without paying due attention to the unique factors that affect the little boy, the nurse may assume that the fear of pain is the major problem, whereas the child may have his own special anxieties not readily identified by an adult. The parents in this instance may be reasonably confident that the child fears being hurt and may therefore confirm that both the knowledge that an injection is needed and the procedure itself are problematic.

King has advocated that nurses working with her model must have knowledge of three dynamic and interacting systems: the personal, the interpersonal and the social. In this context, the nurse will be familiar with the specific nursing and medical activities that contribute to the hospital social system. She will therefore be in a position to predict the circumstances in which the boy might be in need of an injection.

In the second example, a nurse may be caring for a man in his own home who knows that he is dying even though his death is not imminent. His main concern may be to make plans for his ongoing care in the event of his being unable to communicate his wishes at the time. The nurse may have been caring for the man for some time, but he may now want to address this sensitive issue. King recognises that early nurse–patient contact is similar to the meeting of strangers. In this, her work echoes the concerns of Peplau (1952), who also sees the nurse–client relationship as one that develops from a coming together of strangers (see Chapter 10). For this man, the relationship he has with the nurse needs to have moved beyond the meeting of strangers to facilitate further data-gathering concerning his care as he approaches death.

Thus, as the nurse and patient get to know each other better and as the health situation changes, the patient may decide that the time is appropriate for forward planning with respect to the final stages of his life. His fundamental need then will be for care that he may not be able to influence at the time, but his current need is for information to ensure that he understands the care options open to him and for a commitment from the nurse that the care will be of his choosing. In this way, he demonstrates all three of the fundamental health needs identified by King. He needs *information* about what care choices are available and about how to ensure that his wishes for care will be carried out. Such information and its associated activities should help to *prevent* some of the anxiety about his possible loss of autonomy as he becomes increasingly *unable to care* for himself.

Detailed information will be required by the nurse about many aspects of his forthcoming care, and together they will need to consider physical, emotional and possibly spiritual care. The patient will need to set out his expectations about his care if and when he can no longer make his wishes known. The nurse will need to carefully document these expectations because it may be difficult to estimate when the time will come for them to be implemented. Time can distort what is remembered from the nursing history and health assessment, and there may be other nurses involved in the man's care. What is written should be carefully checked for accuracy with the patient as when the data are needed to activate a plan of care, he may not be able to fulfil this role.

Once the data have been gathered and analysed, King recommends compiling a written list of problems in the patient's nursing records. Such a list will often be updated as more is learned about a particular patient. For the little boy, one problem will be his fear of being hurt. Another will be his fear of injections. For the man planning for his future care, the main problem will be how to ensure that his wishes are carried out irrespective of which health care personnel are involved at the time.

Goal list and nursing plan

King values mutual goal-setting in the making of a nursing plan, but this may turn out not to be the case at first for the child in this example. For the nurse, cognisant that some injections are usually needed for a child having a surgical procedure, both to induce anaesthesia and to provide postoperative pain relief, a goal to eliminate or minimise the pain and to gain the child's trust that this can happen may seem appropriate. For the child, the only acceptable goal may be to have no injections at all, and as Thornes (1991: 9) has argued in a recent National Association for the Welfare of Children in Hospital's (NAWCH) publication, 'Every effort should be made to reduce the number of painful or frightening procedures while the child is conscious.'

In this instance, the relevance of King's inclusion of the concept of power in her writings about nursing is pertinent. She argues that 'in any organisation one will see the influence and/or effects of power' (King, 1981: 126). Power is not vested in some people rather than others but is the result of particular interpersonal relationships in a given situation. Nurses are at times in a position of power and may use this power to persuade a patient to accept a goal that the nurse believes is appropriate. Children can sometimes be hard to persuade, especially when they are too young to recognise the distribution of power in a particular social system. However, their autonomy can be respected by listening to their views about treatment options (Brykcznska, 1995). In this example, the child may not be persuaded that minimising or eliminating the pain of injections is adequate. The nurse should then agree a goal for no injections of which the child is aware. Such an approach offers the best chance of the child being content in hospital and bodes well for greater confidence in health care matters as he gets older.

The man who is determined to plan for terminal care of a type that he feels appropriate will have as one goal the adequate and clear communication of his wishes in a way that is as binding as possible on health care staff. He wants the power to influence what happens to him even when he can no longer communicate easily with others. Alongside this will be the goal of achieving high-quality and appropriate care that takes account of his wishes. In agreeing these goals with the patient, the nurse may need to set aside her own ideas about terminal care if they are not entirely congruent with the patient's. She has a responsibility to inform the patient of any concerns she has about the exact nature of care he is requesting, but the decision ultimately rests with him.

Planning will be facilitated by trying to understand the patient's point of view (King, 1989). The involvement of other members of the health care team will often be imperative if goals are to be met. In the example of the child who fears injections, the nurse will need to work closely with the anaesthetist to achieve the desired outcome. If the situation is not unusual and a ward or hospital strategy has previously been developed, the nurse may feel confident with early assurances to the child that alternatives to injections are possible. If this is not the case, the nurse, acting as the child's advocate, will need to talk with the anaesthetist before plans are agreed.

King again promotes patient involvement in care by advocating that the means of goal attainment should be agreed. Recognising that this may be hindered by a lack of knowledge, she emphasises the place of patient education in such a plan. For example, a nurse may often need to introduce patients to the various options available to them before it is possible to agree on actions that might be taken. King recognises that nurses need to remain up to date with developments in the natural and behavioural sciences and with technical advances relevant to nursing in order to fulfil the role of knowledgeable practitioner.

The patient in this example is a child, but the need for education is unchanged even though the method of informing the child of possible options needs tailoring to his developmental stage. When discussions involve possible procedural options, the use of a favourite doll or toy can be helpful to show the child what will take place. Children in hospital can often be seen with bandaged toys, or toys with shields over their eyes as nurses and parents try to find ways of extending their familiarity with what is taking place both to themselves and to other children they might see.

One option for this child might be for anaesthesia to be induced using anaesthetic gases via a face mask. Such an approach has gained increasing popularity of late in both the UK and Canada (Goresky and Muir, 1996). An oral premedication might be planned to further relieve his anxiety. An option for postoperative pain relief, assuming that the use of oral analgesia might not provide adequate pain control, is to insert an intramuscular cannula into the child's thigh while he is anaesthetised. If, following a simple explanation of what these two strategies involve, the child seems happy with the options, the nurse can plan ways of extending his understanding of and familiarity with what will take place. These then will form part of the intervention stage of the care planned. Familiarising a child with what will take place may sometimes occur in the planning stage if, without it, agreement on the way forward cannot be reached.

Planning care with the man being cared for at home and wanting to arrange the details of his future care is likely to be facilitated by the involvement of others. There may be a need to involve someone with a specific knowledge of the current legal position for making plans for care in advance. At the moment, people can make their wishes known through advance directives or living wills, but these are not legally binding on relatives or carers. However, Kennedy and Grubb (1994) advise that health professionals should respect advance directives whenever reasonably possible.

If the patient is agreeable, it will also be important for any close relatives, particularly the man's next of kin, to be included in discussions about his future care. In the event of details contained in any written instructions being difficult or impossible for nurses and other health care personnel to follow, the next of kin will be better able to advise if he or she has been involved from the planning stage and understands the main concerns felt by the man and the principles of care that he believed were important.

During the planning stage, the nurse will make every effort to provide as much information as possible for the man about care options so that he can make an informed choice. This is in keeping with King's emphasis on patient education as a means of producing a realistic and effective plan, and with DiNardo's view that nurses working with King's model can help patients to choose between care alternatives (DiNardo, 1989). As indicated earlier, this period in the man's care episode will be greatly facilitated by the nature of the relationship already developed between the nurse and the patient. For example, it may be necessary for the nurse to explain various possible scenarios that could occur during the terminal stages of the man's life. These may be situations that he has not thought about because he lacks the knowledge and experience of terminal care that the nurse brings to their discussions. Only through a relationship of mutual trust and respect that has already negotiated some challenging care choices, will such difficult issues be addressed successfully.

The planning stage will be complete when the man is content with the written directive he has produced, both in terms of its comprehensiveness with regard to specific terminal care concerns, and of its clarity for those who might be implementing his care plan in the future.

Nursing intervention and the delivery of care

King's concern to promote meaningful interactions, or *transactions*, can be seen with the nurse caring for the child who fears injections. At the planning stage, it was agreed that anaesthesia would be induced through the use of anaesthetic gases administered via a mask and that an intramuscular cannula inserted under anaesthesia would aid the giving of analgesia in the postoperative period. The child should be offered the opportunity to hold a mask, fit it onto his face and try it out on a toy. Playing with a doll already fitted with an intramuscular cannula may help the child to accept this intervention. If the nurse joins in such learning activities with a recognition of their potential not only to inform, but also to give fun and pleasure, her relationship with the little boy will develop. She will be seen as a friend and as a person willing to play, and this may do much to allay anxiety and to promote trust. Play activities such as these, in the presence of and including the parents, will also reinforce for the parents the interventions that they are likely to witness. The greater their familiarity with and confidence about what will take place, the more able they will be to reassure their child.

Accompanying the child to the anaesthetic room and using opportunities to remind him of the early play that took place may also help when the execution of the plan is in part taken over by the anaesthetist and other operating theatre staff. The nurse will be keen to assess how the boy is coping with the procedure but will also want to ensure that any accompanying parent is managing the inevitable stress of seeing the child anaesthetised and then leaving him in the care of others.

It is unusual in most health care settings for plans to be made that require implementation some time in the future. This will, however, be the case for the man being cared for at home. In this example, the man is already at the stage of receiving some nursing care, so any directives are likely to be in operation within, for example, weeks or months. For people who write advanced directives well before any episode of ill-health, there is a need for updating and review so that any instructions can be confidently regarded by carers as a current indication of their wishes.

Interventions that take place for the dying man will need to take note of his written wishes. Ideally, the same nurse(s) who helped to plan his care will look after him as they will have additional insights into the principles of care that he wanted to receive. Care in such situations places an even greater responsibility on health carers, and they will repeatedly need to revisit the man's wishes to ensure that they are carried out. Here, King's concept of power in care situations is again relevant. Once the man is unable to communicate his wishes verbally or non-verbally, nurses need to guard against resuming a role that sees them as empowered to decide afresh on relevant care interventions. In this instance, a nurse must use her power to ensure that the patient's wishes are fulfilled if at all possible.

Progress notes

For the little boy who fears injections, the nurse will be able to record that the goal of no injections was achieved (outcome) but will also want to record how acceptable the process was to the child and his parents. She will note any evidence of stress experienced by the child prior to the operation and his behaviour in the immediate postoperative period.

In particular, she may document the suitability of an intramuscular cannula for pain relief for a child afraid of injections. She will look for evidence of the adequacy of pain relief, probably using a flow chart, in particular whether the method of administration caused any difficulties. Although intramuscular cannulae allow for analgesia to be given into a muscle without using a needle, the procedure may in many ways appear similar to a child. It is conceivable that a child frightened by the thought of an injection might show similar signs of distress when analgesia is offered for administration through a cannula.

Progress notes for the dying man when he cannot communicate readily will be limited to the nurse's own opinions and observations of how well his aims for terminal care have been met and how high a quality of care was achieved. She will also want to involve any other people who know the man well and who were a party to his care-planning. For example, if he particularly wanted to avoid the intervention of having a urinary catheter inserted, the nurse will find it easy to judge whether this was achieved but may find it harder to judge whether this was detrimental to his overall care.

Final summaries may help nurses to begin to evaluate the effectiveness of King's model of nursing in particular situations. It is important to assess the value of the general thrust of King's model compared with the specific concerns of other models. In both of the examples cited in this chapter, the nature of the nurse–patient relationship in the patient's unique care environment was crucial. To achieve the agreed goals, a relationship of considerable trust was needed. In the first example, this needed to develop very rapidly, play being an important element. In the second example, it was the more sustained relationship that allowed for difficult and sensitive care decisions to be effectively addressed. The social emphasis in King's model might therefore be regarded as a very suitable focus in care situations such as those described.

References

Brykczynska, G. (1995) Ethical considerations in child care. In Fatchett, A. (ed.) *Childhood to Adolescence: Caring for Health*. London, Baillière Tindall.

Burney, M.A. (1992) King and Neuman: in search of the nursing paradigm. *Journal of Advanced Nursing*, 17, 601–3.

DiNardo, P.B. (1989) Evaluation of the nursing theory of Imogene M. King. In Riehl-Sisca, J.P. (ed.) *Conceptual Models for Nursing Practice*. Norwalk, CT, Appleton & Lange.

Goresky, G.V. and Muir, J. (1996) Inhalation induction of anaesthesia. *Canadian Journal of Anaesthesia*, 43, 1085–9.

Kennedy, I. and Grubb, A. (1994) *Medical Law*. London, Butterworths.

King, I.M. (1964) Nursing theory – problems and prospect. *Nursing Science*, 17, 27–31.

King, I.M. (1971) *Toward a Theory for Nursing*. New York, John Wiley & Sons.

King, I.M. (1981) *A Theory for Nursing: Systems, Concepts, Process*. New York, John Wiley & Sons.

King, I.M. (1984) *Effectiveness of Nursing Care: Use of a Goal-oriented Nursing Record System in End Stage Renal Disease*. American Association of Nephrology Nurses and Technicians Journal, 11(2): 11–17, 60.

King, I.M. (1986) *Curriculum and Instruction in Nursing*. Norwalk, CT, Appleton-Century-Crofts.

King, I.M. (1989) King's general systems framework and theory. In Riehl-Sisca, J.P. (ed.) *Conceptual Models for Nursing Practice*. Norwalk, CT, Appleton & Lange.

McKenna, H. (1997) *Nursing Theories and Models*. London, Routledge.

Peplau, H. (1952) *Interpersonal Relations in Nursing*. New York, G.P. Putnam & Sons.

Thornes, R. (1991) *Just for the Day*. London, NAWCH.

Weed, L. (1969) *Medical Records, Medical Education and Patient Care*. Cleveland, Case Western Reserve University Press.

Chapter 10 Peplau's development model of nursing

Hildegard Peplau trained as a nurse at Pottsdown Hospital School of Nursing in Pennsylvania and worked subsequently in a range of settings including Bellevue Psychiatric Hospital and, as a member of the US army nurse corps, in a neuropsychiatric hospital in England. She developed and taught the graduate programme in psychiatric nursing, first at Columbia University, New York and subsequently at Rutgers University. Following her retirement in 1974, she continued to be active within the field of psychosocial nursing and has served on numerous committees and advisory councils.

According to Peplau, nursing is a:

significant therapeutic interpersonal process which functions co-operatively with other human processes that make health possible for individuals. (1952: 16)

Her emphasis on the interpersonal nature of nursing identifies the distinctive contribution that nursing can make to health care. It is in the relationships between people that the origins of many nursing problems lie, and it is in the interpersonal domain that interventions have to be made if people are to continue to develop.

Key components of care

The nature of people

Peplau's understanding of people and their needs was much influenced by the work of Harry Stack Sullivan, a psychiatrist writing in the 1940s and early 50s who sought to develop ideas about the human mind first put forward by the psychoanalyst Sigmund Freud. According to Sullivan (1952), most human behaviour is motivated by one of two fundamental drives: the drive for satisfaction and the drive for security. If both of these drives are satisfied, a state of *euphoria* exists, but when one or both are frustrated, tension arises. There are two principal kinds of tension: tension to do with needs and tension to do with anxiety. Need-related tensions arise when the drive for satisfaction is frustrated, whereas anxiety-related tensions arise when the need for security cannot be met.

Tensions are powerful motivators of behaviour. Tensions of anxiety to do with self-esteem, for example, can encourage people to take steps to bolster their self-image in order to reduce the anxiety that they are experiencing. Tensions of need, for example the need for food or the need for contact, motivate behaviour such as eating or getting closer to another person. Sullivan calls these actions that alleviate tensions 'transformations'. Some of these can be relatively obvious and overt, whereas others are more hidden. Phantasy, for example, is a covert way of reducing anxiety and is an important aspect of the person.

Over time, we develop habits or recurrent ways of dealing with the tensions we experience. These are what Sullivan calls 'dynamisms'. They influence the ways in which we relate to one another and help to constitute a 'self-system' whose task it is to manage (and where possible eliminate) anxiety (Figure 10.1).

Fundamental to Sullivan's theory is the idea that much human behaviour is motivated by the need for security. When this security is threatened, anxiety arises, and one of the best ways of dealing with this anxiety is by communicating and establishing meaningful interpersonal relations with others. While this theory was developed primarily for use in therapy, Peplau took many of the basic ideas and developed them for use in nursing.

According to Peplau, people have biological, psychological and social qualities that motivate them towards self-maintenance, reproduction and growth. As in Sullivan's theory, they possess a self-system concerned with the management of anxiety. Biological and psychological insecurities create anxiety. Mild to moderate levels may be easy to cope with, but stronger ones can lead to negative responses such as panic, avoidance, withdrawal and the inability to function effectively. Very occasionally, extreme levels of anxiety can cause *regression*, the person showing behaviours that lack maturity and integration. Growth and development are facilitated by communication and good interpersonal relationships since both of these reduce levels of anxiety.

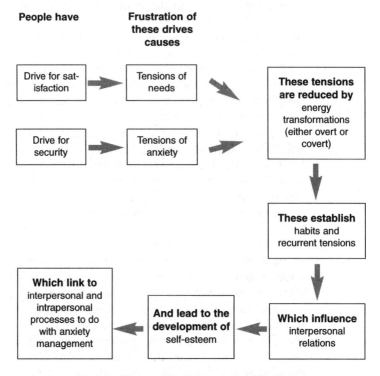

Figure 10.1 Key elements in Sullivan's
theory of human nature

The causes of problems likely to require nursing intervention

The concept of anxiety is a central feature of Peplau's model and problems requiring nursing intervention link mainly to anxiety and worry. Some of the causes of these problems may be physical, such as disease and injury. Others may be psychological and/or social, linking to difficulties in interpersonal relationships. All contribute to the sense of illness that people experience when they require nursing care.

The nature of assessment – orientation

Like a number of nurse theorists writing before the first descriptions of the nursing process, Peplau does not use the term 'assessment' very often in her work. Instead, she talks of nurses and patients passing through an initial *orientation phase* in their relationship. During this, nurses learn more about the difficulties that a patient may be experiencing, and help patients to develop *insight* into the problems that face them. Nurses use their experience and professional insight to help to clarify for patients the source of their difficulties. During this phase also, patients come to learn that the nurse is someone who will participate in their health care.

Peplau recognises that gathering data about patients can be problematic, particularly because so many factors need to be considered. She advocates some form of organisation in the study and collection of data but accepts that 'hunches' (Peplau 1988: 276) may provide a guide. In this, she seems to acknowledge that intuition may play a part in nursing practice, but as a means of influencing further data-gathering rather than as an indication to exploit the relationship or to intervene.

Thus, orientation suggests more than assessment as conventionally defined. While there are similarities in the two stages in that data are gathered, the relationship between the patient and nurse is potentially more equal in orientation than in assessment. There is an emphasis on developing mutual regard and trust, and this in turn should begin to ease any patient tension or anxiety. The orientation phase is thus an important part in building the patient's sense of security.

The nature of planning and goal-setting – identification

Following the orientation phase is the *identification phase*, during which the patient begins to identify the nurse as someone who can help. She encourages the patient to express his feelings about his condition without rejecting anything that is expressed. This way, good interpersonal communication can be encouraged.

During this phase, a nursing diagnosis will be made and a care plan formulated. Patients are involved in the identification of goals to the extent that they provide the evidence that the nurse needs in order to know what these should be.

The focus of nursing intervention during implementation of the care plan – exploitation

As in many nursing models, Peplau's model has little to say about the specific interventions that nurses should make during the *exploitation phase* of their relationship. However, using all the means at her disposal, the nurse will act to alleviate tensions and anxiety, to remove blocks to further development, and to aid personal and interpersonal growth. She may provide access to needed resources, she may counsel, and she may take on the role of others in order to help the patient to develop a better insight into the problems that are being experienced. What Peplau (1969) has called *professional closeness* is an essential part of the nurse–patient relationship at this stage in its development, but throughout the exploitation phase, it is the prime responsibility of the patient to move forward.

In this, the exploitation phase differs from the intervention stage of the nursing process. With all models, intervention will involve the nurse and the patient to some degree, but with Peplau's model the chief action required during the exploitation phase must be carried out by the patient. This is consistent with ideas that see needs being addressed through effective interpersonal relationships. It is usually the patient who must be actively involved in such communications. These may be with nursing or other professional staff or with other people related to the felt need. The nursing role is likely to be one of encouragement and of supplying any necessary resources to the patient. While acknowledging that both nurse and patient develop competencies, Forchuk (1993) sees the development of patient or client competencies as the priority in the therapeutic relationship.

The nature of evaluation – resolution

There is little talk of 'evaluation' in the descriptions of Peplau's model offered by the author herself. Instead, she describes the *resolution phase*, which occurs towards the end of the nurse's relationship with the patient. Here, the patient ceases to identify with the nurse and what she is doing, and the nurse too withdraws from the relationship to reflect on what has been achieved. This phase is significantly different from the evaluation stage of the nursing process, which focuses on judgements about the success or otherwise of particular nursing interventions and the degree to which goals have been met. The nursing process says little about the importance of terminating the nurse's contact and involvement with the patient. In Peplau's model, resolution can, by definition, only occur when the patient is able to be free from nursing assistance and is able to act independently. The completion of the resolution phase will therefore itself be one measure of success of the activities undertaken during all the other phases of the nurse–patient relationship.

The role of the nurse

According to Peplau, the nurse can adopt one of six main roles. She may act as a stranger, the role in which she is first likely to encounter the patient or client. She may also act as a resource person by providing access to the means of resolution and recovery. Alternatively, she may act as a teacher, a leader, a surrogate and a counsellor. In the latter two roles, she has an important job to do in helping the person she is caring for to overcome hurdles to successful development, and in resolving intrapersonal and interpersonal conflicts.

Using Peplau's model

Earlier in this chapter, the significant contribution of the work of Harry Stack Sullivan to the development of Peplau's model was noted. In particular, Sullivan was concerned with security as a motivator of human behaviour and with the anxiety that results if a sense of security is absent. One way of coping with anxiety is through effective interpersonal relationships, and this notion, together with Peplau's belief in the human capacity for development, has formed the main platform for her model.

The two examples in this chapter will therefore be concerned with anxiety related to a loss of security. Deliberately, neither example is hospital based, because much of Peplau's own work gives instances of patients being cared for in hospital. Similarly, she frequently writes about patients whose problems are largely those associated with a particular medical diagnosis. Thus, one example here will consider an adult man with advanced HIV disease whose main concern is a feeling of potential isolation in his own home. The other example explores the difficulties faced by a teenage girl with anxieties about attending school.

Peplau acknowledges that individuals react in different ways when faced with health-related problems. What is similar, however, according to Peplau (1988), is the initial and necessary action taken by the individual to access professional help. She sees two important factors in the beginning of a nurse–patient relationship. First, the individual must recognise, at least to a degree, that a health problem exists. Peplau calls this a 'felt need'. Second, the individual must seek professional help.

These two factors, seen as so important by Peplau, suggest that the use of her model will in practice be limited to those people who both perceive a health need and ask for help. Thus, individuals who fail to recognise an existing health problem, do not want professional help or cannot communicate verbally might not be best served by this model. Similarly, these factors would seem to exclude Peplau's model from use in preventive care.

As stated earlier, Peplau describes four stages, or phases, in the nurse–patient relationship: orientation, identification, exploitation and resolution. She sees these phases as both interlocking and overlapping, and she identifies different tasks and roles for the nurse at each phase. While these four phases may at first sight look similar to the stages of nursing process, they differ in a number of ways. As the two examples in this chapter develop through the use of these four special phases, some mention will be made of how each differs from the largely parallel stage of the nursing process.

Orientation

During this phase, when the nurse and patient meet as strangers, the nurse aims to familiarise the patient with the nursing knowledge and skills available to address his or her perceived health need. The health need itself may be clarified and further defined. The nurse also aims to engender sufficient trust in her relationship with the patient that the second phase, identification, can be embarked on with the patient's full cooperation and willingness.

In the first example, the community nurse meets the man with advanced HIV disease in his own home. He is becoming increasingly unwell, believes that most of his close neighbours are unaware of his health status, and fears their reaction to him as his physical limitations increase. He lives with his male partner, but they have never felt particularly welcome at local gatherings. Another friend who died of HIV disease was ostracised and ignored by neighbours once his diagnosis was known. The man's anxiety is such that he wonders how he will cope with spending more time at home in a progressively weak state.

During the orientation phase, the nurse and the man will get to know each other and will further define his felt need. The nurse will want to find out exactly what threat he perceives to his security and how the resultant anxiety is experienced. He may describe things that previously happened to his friend, for example verbal abuse from neighbours or graffiti (related to gay men and AIDS) daubed on his property. He may identify that he feels inhibited to leave his home and sleeps poorly at night. Ryan Belcher and Brittain Fish (1995) recognise the importance in Peplau's model of exploring events that precede a current health situation, and the nurse will encourage the man to clarify the nature of his existing relationship with his neighbours. This may help to put his concerns into context.

It will also be important for the nurse to be non-judgemental (McCann, 1997) and to show genuine positive regard for the man if she is to gain his trust and offer him meaningful help. 'Nursing symbolizes acceptance of people as they are', wrote Peplau (1988: 31). She will need to be explicit about her own knowledge and skills with regard to both HIV disease and community liaison. The man's body language may further point to his level of anxiety, and the nurse may hope for a more relaxed appearance as the orientation phase progresses. Orientation interlocks and overlaps with the other phases of Peplau's system for implementing her model. Where the nurse's own reaction to the patient and his trust in her positive regard is so critical, the orientation phase may be lengthy and may certainly overlap with identification. Simpson (1991) also found that significant time was needed to develop a therapeutic relationship.

The teenage girl who dislikes attending school may have experienced difficulties for some time. She may seek help from the school nurse once she perceives the problem as one that requires professional help and if she regards the nurse as an appropriate confidante. Commonly, the concerns that lead to loss of a sense of security are ones difficult to describe to someone else. This can be exacerbated if the available professional seems remote or unlikely to identify with the difficulty.

As Peplau acknowledges, nurses can assume many different roles, and the school nurse in particular needs to be someone whom young people can trust and with whom they feel at ease.

During the orientation phase, the nurse will ask about events that have led to the girl's anxiety. In this example, the girl may demonstrate a willingness to develop her understanding of what is happening. Peplau (1988: 20) cites questions such as 'What is wrong with me?' 'Why should this thing happen to me?' as evidence of a desire for a greater insight into the meaning of experiences. It may become clear that the girl is convinced that she is not going to gain the grades adequate for entry into the sixth form. She may describe her parents' wish that she studies hard but add to this her own belief that she is not academically able enough. Attendance at school may continually convince her that high grades are beyond her reach, and, to avoid the resultant anxiety, she may choose to be absent.

As the orientation phase develops and the girl and school nurse move beyond the role of strangers within the relationship, the nurse may seek to extend the girl's understanding of her need for help. For example, she will want to explore fully both the felt need for absence from school to relieve anxiety as well as the way this further disadvantages the girl in the pursuit of adequate grades. She will also ask about past successes at school and about the girl's relationship with staff members, which Coleman (1992) sees as being very important. The nurse may try to access what exactly has led to the girl's poor opinion of her own abilities and may discover that a particular teacher has been openly pessimistic about her chances of success.

It will be important during this phase that the nurse is honest about her knowledge and skills. She can identify to the girl that she can probably help her to manage the situation so that she will feel less anxious and more secure. She must also confirm that she has no remit to influence examination results nor can she contribute directly to the girl's academic skills.

Identification

During the identification phase, the patient begins to identify the nurse as someone able to help. At this time, some patients will take a more active role than others in planning to alleviate their problems. Peplau sees such patients sharing in the nurse's optimism and cheerfulness about the prospects for problems to be solved and thus sees them as having some control. As the nurse–patient relationship develops in the identification phase, the patient is helped to see ways in which he can take further control of what is happening to him. He may learn new strategies and behaviours to respond more appropriately to events in his current situation.

For the man with HIV disease, the nurse will want to develop his ability to respond to the threats he perceives exist. She may initially try to help him disentangle what happened to his friend from the reality of his own experience. There will be a need to be 'straightforward' (Peplau 1988: 36) in the nurse's questioning if she is to understand the true nature of his concerns. She will want to explore in some depth what kind of interpersonal relationships exist between the man, his partner and their immediate neighbours. She may discover that reticence to form friendships is a product of the man's own lack of security. There may be little in the neighbours' behaviour to support his concerns. On the other hand, and within the developing therapeutic relationship, the man may feel empowered to tell the nurse of episodes of homophobia that have undermined his confidence in making approaches to certain local people.

During identification, therefore, greater clarity is achieved about the felt need and about the patient's preconceptions and expectations. In this example, it will be important to ascertain whether the patient is paying more attention to his friend's experience or to the reality of his own circumstances. The nurse will also develop a clearer idea about the patient's existing interpersonal skills and how they might be used in the current situation. She will try to show him different ways in which he might respond, because one aim of the identification phase is for the patient to develop confidence in his ability to deal successfully with his own problems.

Identification thus differs from planning and goal-setting within the nursing process. Certainly, the way forward into the exploitation phase will be addressed and the respective roles of the nurse and patient clarified. However, this is unlikely to produce a series of easily measurable goals with specific nursing and patient inputs listed.

If, at orientation, the relationship between the teenage girl and the school nurse has developed into one of trust, the girl may, during identification, be able to express and explore feelings that she has previously kept to herself. Peplau sees identification as providing an opportunity for the expression of feelings that might be disapproved of within a particular culture. Here, the girl might talk of considerable anger at the pressure she feels from her parents. Within the nurse–patient relationship, she may vent feelings that others might not understand. This has the two-fold benefit of relieving some of her anger and anxiety, and of helping the nurse to understand her better.

As the period of identification proceeds, the nurse and the girl will need to clarify what each expects of the other as their relationship develops. In this situation, they may agree that the girl has the main role in trying to explain her difficulties to her parents, while the nurse may take the lead in negotiations within the school.

Exploitation

It is during this important phase that the patient moves beyond receiving help from the nurse and other professionals and begins to translate their help into effective personal action. By this time in the nurse–patient relationship, the patient should be fully aware of what help has been and can be offered and should be able to selectively put what he has learned to useful effect in his own interests.

Depending on the decisions agreed during the identification phase, the man concerned about his relations with his neighbours may be encouraged by the nurse to try to establish a more meaningful contact with them. If, however, his anxieties stem from real instances of homophobia that seriously threaten his sense of security, the nurse and other community workers may be his most valuable resources in trying to alter existing attitudes among his neighbours. In a rather different context, Peplau describes this balance in the exploitation phase between a need for the patient to be dependent and a need for him to be independent.

During the exploitation phase, therefore, the nurse may take on a number of roles identified by Peplau. If the man is to attempt to develop improved and more open relationships with his neighbours, he may need the nurse to be both teacher and counsellor. As a counsellor, the nurse may help the man to redefine the behaviour of his neighbours in a more positive way. As a teacher, she may then assist in the extension of his interpersonal skills so that he and his neighbours may come to know and understand each other better. If, however, the man has genuine cause to feel threatened, the nurse may adopt the challenging role of surrogate to try to resolve the interpersonal conflict. In this, she will need to help both the patient and his neighbours to understand the similarities and differences that exist between individuals, and she will hope to be given the opportunity to explore more appropriate local responses to the concerns felt. For the patient, she may be seen in a surrogate mother role and therefore as someone acceptable to consult and negotiate on his behalf.

A community nurse who works regularly in a particular area may be best placed to tackle such complex issues through her contact with local people and their trust in her abilities and motives. She may already attend meetings on current concerns with other community workers and may enlist their support to increase public awareness of the needs of individuals with health problems. She may highlight the particular problems of alienation that can accompany a diagnosis of HIV disease (Anderson, 1992). There may be a local newsletter in which similar issues can be aired, and the nurse may also decide to arrange for delivery of information leaflets about HIV to homes in the neighbourhood. With the man's consent, she may talk directly to certain close neighbours to try to ease their relations with the man and his partner. Again, her knowledge of local people may enable her to select one or two key individuals whom she knows will be able positively to influence the responses of others to the man, his sexual orientation and his current health problem.

In the case of the teenage girl, having learned what help the nurse can offer, she may begin to make use of her abilities. In order to confront her parents about her unhappiness and fears, the girl may rehearse how she might begin. She might spend time with the nurse in an environment where she can practise without embarrassment. The nurse may ask her to imagine the responses her parents might give and to plan how she might respond without losing her temper. There may also be the opportunity at such a rehearsal for the nurse to put forward alternative responses that the parents might make and for the girl to be encouraged to mentally put herself in their situation.

The nurse may take the lead in trying to ascertain from the school the expected achievements of the girl. She might identify those members of staff who feel able to offer her additional help and support. She may discover that the real cause of the girl's repeated absences has not been understood by the teachers and that once they are informed, they have ideas about how to help her themselves.

As such relationships develop, it may become clear whether the girl has misjudged her own abilities and chances of success or whether her self-assessment is accurate. Further activity in the exploitation phase will be largely dependent on this. For example, if the girl's assessment is generally accurate, she will need help to build up her feelings of self-worth by focusing on things she is good at and in which she has skills. Meetings between teachers and the family may go some way towards exploring meaningful opportunities other than further academic study.

Resolution

The challenge offered by Peplau's model to sets of medical ideas is exemplified in her elaboration of what constitutes resolution. She argues that resolution is not just when a medical problem is resolved or when, for example, sutures are removed from a wound, because such recovery may not coincide with the patient's wish or readiness to terminate the nurse–patient relationship. For nurses working with this model, resolution is instead 'the gradual freeing from identification with helping persons and the generation and strengthening of ability to stand more or less alone' (Peplau 1988: 40).

Resolution will occur for the man with HIV disease when he no longer feels threatened by his neighbours and when he feels confident to continue to develop his interpersonal relationships locally without the support of the nurse. Signs that this stage has been reached may include his increased willingness to leave his house and his reporting an improved sleep pattern. In addition, he may contact the nurse less frequently and may require less of her time at each visit. He may describe events that have reassured him concerning his neighbours' attitudes towards him. A situation of great intimacy was never sought, so events that confirm a lack of threat will be sufficient to ease his anxiety.

Resolution for the teenage girl may be signalled when she returns to school on a regular basis. However, because resolution is about the person or patient feeling confident for the nurse–patient relationship to terminate, it may end when the girl feels that her relations with her parents and with the staff are such that negotiations and plans can proceed in the absence of the nurse. Meetings at which she initially needed the nurse's personal support may start to occur without her. Peplau's model sees interpersonal relations as a means to individual development, and this can occur even when problems have still to be fully solved.

As has been shown, Peplau's model is largely about adults using interpersonal skills to remove feelings of anxiety and to increase a sense of security. During this process, development takes place for the nurse and the patient, and, as the nurse works with the patient, she becomes increasingly effective (Ryan Belcher and Brittain Fish, 1995). The model has been used extensively in mental health nursing. What has been demonstrated in this chapter is that the model, while not being appropriate in all care settings, does have things to offer in many situations where relationships are crucial to the patient's needs. It may nevertheless be a difficult and inappropriate model to implement when planned nurse–patient contact is short. Simpson (1991), for example, has questioned its use with patients being admitted to hospital for 48 hours or less.

References

Anderson, C. (1992) Living with HIV. In Anderson, C. and Wilkie, P. (eds) *Reflective Helping in HIV and AIDS.* Buckingham, Open University Press.

Belcher, J. Ryan and Brittain Fish, L.J. (1995) Hildegard E. Peplau. In George, J.B. (ed.) *Nursing Theories: The Base for Professional Nursing Practice.* London, Prentice-Hall International.

Coleman, J.C. (ed.) (1992) *The School Years: Current Issues in the Socialisation of Young People.* London, Routledge.

Forchuk, C. (1993) *Hildegard E. Peplau: Interpersonal Nursing Theory.* London, Sage.

McCann, T.V. (1997) Willingness to provide care and treatment for patients with HIV/AIDS. *Journal of Advanced Nursing,* 25, 1033–9.

Peplau, H.E. (1952) *Interpersonal Relations in Nursing.* New York, Putnam's Sons.

Peplau, H.E. (1969) Professional closeness. *Nursing Forum*, 4, 342–60.

Peplau, H.E. (1988) *Interpersonal Relations in Nursing*. Basingstoke, Macmillan Education.

Simpson, H. (1991) *Peplau's Model in Action*. Basingstoke, Macmillan.

Sullivan, H.S. (1952) *The Interpersonal Theory of Psychiatry*. New York, Norton.

Chapter 11 Neuman's systems model of nursing

In this chapter, we will look closely at a nursing model that has been used across a wide range of nursing situations and that is likely to be familiar to many nurses working in the UK – the systems model of nursing developed by Betty Neuman. In contrast to some of the models discussed elsewhere in this book, Neuman's approach does not encourage us to see people as biological systems, as organisms at a particular stage in development or as part of an interaction process. Instead, people are perhaps best understood as *open systems* in interaction with their environments.

Betty Neuman trained as a nurse in the 1940s at People's Hospital School of Nursing in Akron, Ohio before working as a hospital nurse, a school nurse and an industrial nurse in California. After a period of time as a clinical teacher, Neuman worked to promote nursing involvement in mental health and was a key player in the establishment of nurse counsellors within Los Angeles community crisis centres. It was as a teacher at the University of California, Los Angeles that she first developed her nursing model as part of the effort to extend nursing beyond the medical model. After returning to Ohio, she has continued to work as a consultant and private practice therapist.

Neuman identifies a range of factors as influencing the development of her model of nursing. These include Hans Selye's (1950) important work on stress and defences against it, as well as more general work in the field of public health identifying important distinctions between primary, secondary and tertiary prevention. Whereas primary prevention is concerned with minimising the risk of disease, secondary and tertiary prevention link more closely to restoring health in those who are sick, and maximising the health potential of those who are chronically or terminally ill, respectively. For Neuman, all these different kinds of prevention are important, and nurses have a unique contribution to make to each of them.

Key components of care

The nature of people

According to Neuman, people have a number of physiological, psychological, socio-cultural and developmental qualities. These qualities between them contribute to a set of *survival factors* unique to that person but which operate within a range of values shared with other individuals. These survival factors include mechanisms regulating body temperature, the strengths and weaknesses of various body parts and ego structure.

A person's core structure of survival factors, or *basic structure*, is protected by a number of internal *lines of resistance*. These help to establish a *normal line of defence*, or state of adaptation, which the individual is able to maintain over time. Beyond this, however, people are protected by a *flexible line of defence* (sometimes called a flexible line of resistance), which acts as a buffer to prevent stressors breaking through the normal line of defence. The strength of this flexible line of defence fluctuates, however, and lack of sleep, malnutrition and a number of stressors working together can weaken it considerably (Figure 11.1).

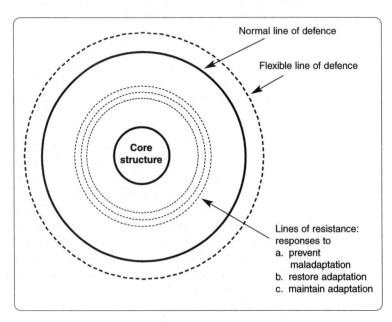

Figure 11.1   Neuman's view of the person

Within each person, five *variable areas* or aspects of the person are defined: the physiological, the psychological, the socio-cultural, the developmental and the spiritual. Each of these may be more or less developed in the case of an individual, and each potentiates behaviour of varying kinds and different styles. Neuman also describes what she calls the *internal environment*, which is established by the boundaries of a particular client/client system; the *external environment*, which consists of the forces and influences external to a particular client/client system; and the *created environment*, which is an 'unconscious mobilisation of all system variables... toward system integration, stability and integrity... its function is to offer a protective coping shield or safe arena for system function' (Neuman, 1995: 31).

The causes of problems likely to require intervention

Three broad types of stress can be experienced:

1. Stress resulting from intrapersonal factors
2. Stress linked to interpersonal processes
3. Stress from extrapersonal factors (for example life circumstances) over which an individual may have little direct control.

Whenever stress is experienced, people *react*, and reaction is usually followed by a process of *reconstitution* as the person returns to a state of relative wellness.

Nursing is called for when the cushioning provided by the flexible line of defence can no longer protect against a stressor or combination of stressors. In these circumstances, the stressor (or stressors) break through the normal line of defence, causing disequilibrium as the lines of resistance surrounding the central core attempt to restore balance. The circumstances in which disequilibrium occurs will vary between individuals (some being very resilient whereas others are not) and depend upon the physiological, psychological, socio-cultural, developmental and spiritual aspects of an individual's make-up.

The nature of assessment – nursing diagnosis and variance from wellness

For nurses working with Neuman's model, assessment involves looking at the potential and actual stressors affecting the individual. This is facilitated by the use of an assessment tool such as the Neuman Nursing Process Format (Neuman, 1995). Using this device, the nurse examines in turn factors relevant to primary, secondary and tertiary prevention.

With respect to primary prevention, risks and possible hazards should be looked for, along with the meanings these have for the patient, lifestyle factors and past coping patterns. With respect to secondary prevention, assessment should look at the reactions that there have been to stressors and the internal and external resources available to resist these reactions. Assessment for tertiary prevention will need to examine the degree of stability following treatment as well as the presence of factors that may lead to possible regression. Both of these latter sources of information can be used to identify appropriate further reconstitution levels (Neuman, 1995).

Throughout assessment, the nurse should seek to identify whether the major sources of stress are intrapersonal, interpersonal or extrapersonal. She should also try to reconcile any differences of perspective between herself and the patient.

The nature of planning and goal-setting – goal identification

Following assessment, goals, along with appropriate intervention strategies, are negotiated between the nurse and patient. If the nurse is mainly concerned with primary prevention, goals should relate to the prevention of maladaptation. When secondary prevention is of greater priority, goals should seek to restore adaptation. When tertiary prevention is the focus, goals should be concerned with maintaining adaptation.

Neuman recommends that nurses distinguish carefully between immediate, intermediate and future goals, and recommends that goals be written in such a way that they specify observable and measurable outcomes. She also recommends the ranking of goals in terms of their importance.

The focus of intervention during the implementation of the care plan – intervention

According to Neuman, intervention can occur whenever a stressor is suspected or identified. More than most other models, Neuman's framework makes explicit the distinctions between primary, secondary and tertiary prevention. Primary prevention, in which Neuman includes the goal of health promotion (Neuman, 1995), aims to protect the normal line of defence and enhance the flexible line of defence. It does this by identifying what is likely to cause stress for an individual and trying to allay it. For those already experiencing stress-related difficulties, secondary prevention aims to strengthen their flexible line of defence. Tertiary prevention, according to Neuman, follows successful secondary prevention and focuses on maintaining adaptation by mobilising an individual's energy resources. Much tertiary prevention uses education as a means of strengthening an individual's resistance to known risk factors.

The nature of evaluation – evaluation of outcomes

For Neuman, the primary goal of nursing is the attainment and maintenance of the client's system stability. To bring this about, nurses may assist and educate individuals, groups and families, and they may intervene to reduce stress factors and the adverse conditions causing these. Overall evaluation of the model therefore involves assessing the extent to which system stability has been restored following nursing intervention. In the shorter term, however, other kinds of evaluation may take place.

For example, Neuman's model distinguishes between short-term and long-term goal outcomes (Neuman, 1995). The former relate to the immediate goals negotiated between the nurse and patient, whereas the latter relate to the future goals that were set, as well as to any immediate goals that were reformulated following feedback on short-term goal outcomes. For nurses working with the model, therefore, ongoing evaluation is likely to examine the extent to which short-term and long-term goal outcomes are being achieved, as well as the appropriateness of corrective action in cases where they are not.

The role of the nurse

A crucial aspect of the nurse's role when working with the Neuman model is the need to remain sensitive to patients' perceptions of their needs and what is happening to them. Perceptual differences between nurse and patient need to be resolved before a care plan is produced, and nurses cannot impose their judgements on others (Venable, 1980). This suggests a role of greater equality with patients than has traditionally been the case.

Using Neuman's model

Neuman's systems model stresses the importance of the relationship between people and their environments. It focuses on stress and the defence mechanisms or survival factors that individuals possess to enable them to cope with the stressors in their lives. Such mechanisms can be biological, psychological, socio-cultural or developmental in character. It is generally when these defence mechanisms are inadequate for the stress being experienced that there is a need for nursing, nursing intervention aiming to preserve or re-establish client system stability.

Of the two examples we will consider in this chapter, one will focus on stress being experienced by a young woman in her twenties who seeks assistance from a nurse at her local health centre. The other will explore the concerns of a recently retired man who is becoming increasingly breathless on exertion and who is referred by his GP to a health visitor whose remit includes addressing the needs of middle-aged and older people. The choice of examples does not indicate that Neuman's model is inappropriate in an inpatient setting. Instead, they are selected in an acknowledgement of the model's development in the field of public health and in recognition of the increasing diversity of health-related problems seen in the community.

Neuman (1989, 1995) advocates the Neuman Nursing Process Format to complement the use of her model. In this, the first stage is concerned with formulating a nursing diagnosis, central to this being determining variance from wellness. Once this has been achieved, goals are identified and interventions undertaken. Finally, an evaluation of outcomes takes place. The stages of Neuman's Format are therefore very similar to those of the nursing process.

Nursing diagnosis and variance from wellness

To achieve a nursing diagnosis and to determine the variance from wellness, the nurse takes a history and analyses the data obtained. Neuman (1995) recommends that the meaning of any stressor identified during the data-gathering stage be validated by both client and nurse. This means that the perceptions of the client and of the nurse about what is happening need to be made apparent. Optimal care-planning can only be achieved, according to Neuman, when the client's perceptions have been clarified. Therefore, the major data-gathering method to be used with Neuman's model is the interview.

In the first example, a young woman of Indian descent but brought up in the UK attends her local health centre initially to ask advice about travel vaccinations. She tells the white, Caucasian practice nurse that her proposed trip to India has been planned by her parents so that a husband can be selected for her. She expects to remain in India after her marriage. She expresses concern about the visit and asks the nurse whether she can talk to her about how she feels. This discussion may need to take place at a later date, but an agreement to listen to her concerns should reassure the girl that her request has been accepted and meet her immediate goal of having someone to talk to outside her family.

According to George (1995), the database needs to be comprehensive enough to determine the existing state of wellness and the actual or potential response to stressors in the person's environment. To this end, the nurse may seek information about the girl's family life and may in particular ask about any other tensions that have arisen as a result of cultural differences. She may ask how earlier difficulties have been resolved and what particular strategies have proved successful. Neuman (1995) has argued that a knowledge of past coping patterns makes it easier to predict what may or may not be accomplished in the present situation. The nurse may learn that the young woman's upbringing has been strict by Western standards and that her social life in particular has been closely controlled by her parents, although she does have a few friends from different cultures. It may become clear that the girl has been unsuccessful in the past in gaining much relaxation of her parents' social rules.

Background information such as biographical data is also seen as helpful by Neuman. The nurse may want to know about the make-up of the girl's immediate family and about those of her extended family also living in the UK. She may discover that the girl is an only child but that her father's brother and his family are also resident in this country. The nurse will hope to gain some understanding about the relationships between the various family members and about the cultural norms that pertain. She may be made aware that although the young woman was born in the UK, the lives of her family and her extended family remain influenced by traditional Hindu beliefs.

In such a situation, namely a nurse from one culture being asked for assistance by someone from a different culture, the importance of sharing perceptions about what is happening is crucial. The practice nurse will want to understand what tensions the proposed trip cause for the young woman and must not assume that her own opinions about arranged marriages, which may well be negative, are the same as the girl's. She may discover that, despite reservations about the idea of having a husband selected for her, the girl is prepared to accept that this is what will happen. On the other hand, the girl may be totally opposed to the idea but feel powerless to do anything about it. The degree of tension being experienced will vary accordingly, as will the focus of care.

Neuman advocates a clear statement of the nursing diagnosis once any perceptual differences between the client and nurse have been resolved. In this example, a statement might acknowledge the rigidity of the family system within which the girl lives and identify the proposed trip as an actual stressor with the potential to breach her flexible line of defence.

In the second example, a man in his late fifties has been referred to a health visitor by his GP because he has experienced some shortness of breath when walking uphill and when gardening. His doctor is treating him for mild heart failure and is also concerned that he smokes heavily. The man has expressed a wish to be helped to give up smoking.

When the health visitor meets the man, she is concerned to find out about his shortness of breath and about his smoking habits. In keeping with Neuman's model, she will be interested in his perception of the problem with his breathing and his view about smoking. She may discover that he regards himself as generally very fit and that the recent limitations to his normal activities are causing him considerable stress because he cannot pursue his favourite activities of walking and gardening as he once could. He may indicate that he has tried in the past to reduce the number of cigarettes he smokes, with little, and only short-term, success.

It will be important for the health visitor to understand what smoking means to the client and what his perception is of his previous attempts to give up. She may find that he has on earlier occasions been encouraged by family and friends to give up smoking despite his state of wellness and lack of any apparent health problems. Now, he may feel more motivated to reduce the number of cigarettes he smokes each day because his chosen activities are being threatened.

The health visitor will also want to gather data about the resources he perceives as being available to help him reduce his tobacco consumption. He may cite his own new-found motivation as the key resource he possesses, as well as the fact that his wife is very supportive and keen for him to give up smoking. He may feel that, since retirement, his life is generally less stressful and that his need for tobacco has consequently reduced. However, he may also identify his previous failure to maintain a reduction in his tobacco use as a major concern and stressor.

The nursing diagnosis will identify that the man has an actual variance from wellness, with physical symptoms of shortness of breath. Smoking is one stressor that has breached his flexible line of defence to produce his symptoms of breathlessness. The other stressors to the client system are the limitations to his favourite activities and the perceived difficulty of giving up smoking.

Goal identification

Neuman (1995) recommends intervention even when a client is not currently reacting adversely to the factors affecting the situation but is deemed to be at risk. This is primary prevention, and in this example the nurse is likely to be concerned that the girl's normal and flexible lines of defence be strengthened to protect her from potential instability. At data-gathering, it was clear that her relationship with her parents is of paramount importance and that, while having reservations about arranged marriages, she also values the traditional customs of her religion. To this end, she is prepared to travel to India in order for her parents to select a husband for her, even though this is not something that she finds easy to accept. While this may be very difficult for the nurse to understand, her role is to help the client to achieve her personal goals.

Neuman mentions immediate, intermediate and future goals. In the case of the young Hindu woman, the goals are likely to be intermediate and future in nature. The girl's goals might include conserving her energy by developing as positive an attitude as possible to the forthcoming trip (intermediate). In this way, her lines of defence will be more effective in protecting her from the stresses that may be encountered when she meets a possible marriage partner (future). She may want to begin the process of disengaging from her friends in this country as she prepares to live in India (intermediate).

In the second example, the man may be very clear what his goals are. For him, the major concern, and therefore his future goal, is to resume his various favourite activities as quickly as possible. To this end, he may now want to give up cigarettes totally rather than reduce the number he smokes (immediate), and maintain this no-smoking stance indefinitely (intermediate and future).

The health visitor is therefore looking to intervene through secondary prevention to improve his variance from wellness (shortness of breath) by helping him to give up smoking. She may also plan to reduce the perceived stress of stopping smoking in order to strengthen the man's flexible line of defence. To this end, she may negotiate with him a goal concerned with coping with any symptoms of nicotine withdrawal.

Together, the client and health visitor will need to decide whether or not some immediate action is required to ease the tension caused by the limitations to the man's normal activities. He will need to consider whether he is prepared to wait until his state of wellness has improved sufficiently for him to resume activities or whether he wants to explore alternative, less strenuous ways of spending his time. It may be that he can continue with enough light gardening and short walks to satisfy his needs in the short term.

Intervention

As has been stated in other chapters, a model of nursing cannot and should not provide detailed strategies for nursing interventions. Instead, it should offer principles or general types of intervention in keeping with the model's philosophy. In this way, nurses can use up-to-date, evidence-based practices suitable to the model to help clients to achieve their goals. Neuman (1995) describes a number of possible nursing actions in relation to primary, secondary and tertiary prevention. For example, she advocates providing information, supporting positive coping, motivating clients towards wellness and educating clients.

The initial intervention by the practice nurse was to support the girl's efforts towards positive coping by spending time with her to discuss her concerns about her forthcoming journey to India. To address the intermediate goals of developing a more positive outlook on the planned trip and its probable consequences, and of beginning the process of disengagement in this country, other strategies will be required. In this instance, it may prove useful that the cultural backgrounds of the nurse and client are so different.

One strategy for developing a positive attitude might be for the girl to explain the importance of family life in her own culture to the nurse. To achieve this, it will be the client who takes on the role of educator. She might be encouraged to high-light to the nurse all the things she finds most positive about her home life and the reasons why these have led her to agree to an arranged marriage. She may be able to describe other family traditions that seem strange to the nurse but with which she feels comfortable. Such a rehearsal of those things she finds of value may serve to bolster her flexible line of defence so that the stres-sors related to the planned trip and marriage will not penetrate or disturb her normal stable state.

Interventions to help the young woman to disengage from friends in this country may be difficult to achieve without threats to her other goal of developing a positive view about what is planned for her. It is probable that some of her Western friends find the notion of an arranged marriage difficult to understand. There may be some goal conflict in the girl exposing herself to possible persuasion by her friends to defy her parents' wishes. Neuman advocates protection of the person (client system) as a means of maintaining system stability, and the nurse might suggest that too much time spent discussing her future with her Western friends might pose an additional system threat.

Nevertheless, the nurse and the client will need to explore the various ways in which the girl can say her goodbyes to her friends without experiencing undue stress. Given the restrictions on her social life, ways are also needed that will not produce conflict with her parents. A compromise may need to be achieved between a social gathering of which her parents might not approve and no opportunity to disengage. Together, the nurse and client might explore the involvement of either a member of the girl's extended family who has sympathy with her difficulty or of a close friend who understands the constraints under which she can act.

Information-giving and education will be key intervention strategies for the middle-aged man with breathing difficulties who wants to stop smoking. However, the necessarily limited and intermittent client–health visitor contact provides a challenge in terms of information-giving and education. Leaflets can be invaluable in bridging the inevitable gap between visits and in giving the client accurate and up-to-date information that he can keep. The suitability of any particular leaflet for a client needs to be established, and the health visitor will want to discuss the contents with the man before leaving it with him.

As stated earlier, Neuman also sees nurses intervening to help people to feel motivated towards achieving a state of improved wellness. In this instance, the man already appears to be highly motivated so the health visitor will be keen to monitor and maintain this, especially as the period of intervention may be lengthy, with the potential for his motivation to waver at times. The health visitor may suggest that a diary is kept for the man to note down both how he is feeling and what coping methods help when he feels the urge to have a cigarette.

As time goes on, the diary should begin to reflect improvements in the man's breathing, and this may further support him throughout the period of care. Ewles and Simnett (1995), among others, have advocated the use of diaries in health promotion. The health visitor might suggest the periodic measurement and recording of the man's peak flow as an additional motivator.

Self-motivation to stop smoking is extremely important as it avoids the client feeling alienated from health care professionals who might otherwise be regarded as dictating a need for a lifestyle change (Blackburn, 1993). Additionally, the long-term nature of the goal to give up smoking requires considerable self-motivation. Even at the beginning of the process, the amount of time that the health visitor can spend with the client will be relatively short and, in this example, she will want to involve the client's wife in the process of intervention as she will be in a position to offer support and encouragement more frequently.

Evaluation of outcomes

Neuman does not write in detail about outcomes other than to indicate that they are achieved by primary, secondary or tertiary prevention and that they are evaluated by reference to the previously set goals. Nurses working with this model will therefore need carefully to consider what methods of evaluation are best suited to its overall philosophy and to the individual client. Given the close association between data-gathering and evaluative methods in most models, it is probable that the interview will often be crucial in evaluating nursing outcomes with Neuman's model.

For the young Hindu woman, the process of evaluation, while important, may seem rather superficial. The client–nurse relationship in this example has focused on a discussion of possible primary prevention strategies both to protect the client's system stability and to strengthen her lines of defence. She may or may not return to see the practice nurse again, although this would be desirable in terms of assessing the value of the nurse's input. It may be that evaluation can only go as far as asking the girl how she feels about the proposed strategies. She may express increased confidence in her ability to prepare for her trip to India, and she may feel that she has a way forward to disengage from relationships in this country. However, the reality may be that the nurse will never know in any more detail how successful she was in helping the girl to face a different and challenging future.

Such a situation, one in which the evaluation of nursing outcomes is difficult to achieve, reinforces the need for nurses working with a particular model to implement it with a number of different patients/clients over a period of time before making judgements about its usefulness in practice. For instance, in the second example included in this chapter, the evaluation of nursing outcomes is not quite as challenging as in the first case, and uses a variety of methods.

Thus, for the man wanting to stop smoking and resume activities such as gardening and walking, different evaluative strategies can be adopted. The health visitor will initially want his opinion on the acceptability of the planned interventions, but later measurements, such as peak flow readings, the number of days since he has had a cigarette and subjective judgements about his breathing when taking exercise, may all be helpful. He may be able to identify that he is walking further or up a steeper gradient without feeling breathless. There may also be outcomes related to feelings of withdrawal and any coping methods that have helped, such as particular foods or nicotine replacement.

References

Blackburn, C. (1993) Gender, class and smoking. *Health Visitor*, 66, 83–5.

Ewles, L. and Simnett, I. (1995) *Promoting Health: A Practical Guide.* Harrow, Scutari Press.

George, J.B. (ed.) (1995) *Nursing Theories: The Base for Professional Nursing Practice.* Norwalk, CT, Appleton & Lange.

Neuman, B. (1989) The Neuman nursing process format: a family case study. In Riehl-Sisca, J.P. (ed.) *Conceptual Models for Nursing Practice,* 3rd edn. Norwalk, CT, Appleton-Century-Crofts.

Neuman, B. (1995) *The Neuman Systems Model.* Norwalk, CT, Appleton & Lange.

Selye, H. (1950) *The Physiology and Pathology of Exposure to Stress.* Montreal, ACTA.

Venable, J.F. (1980) The Neuman health-care systems model: an analysis. In Riehl, J.P. and Roy, C. (eds) *Conceptual Models for Nursing Practice.* Norwalk, CT, Appleton-Century-Crofts.

Chapter 12 Riehl's interaction model of nursing

Joan Riehl's (later Riehl-Sisca) education and training as a nurse took place at the University of Illinois in Urbana and in Chicago. She subsequently worked as a clinical instructor and in-service director in Texas and in California before receiving a Master's degree in nursing from the University of California, Los Angeles (UCLA). After teaching paediatric nursing for a time at California State University, she joined the nursing faculty at UCLA, where she became interested in the development of nursing theory, particularly in the contribution of *symbolic interactionism* to the understanding of people and their responses to health and illness. She has subsequently worked in Texas and Pennsylvania.

In contrast to some of the other models of nursing that we have considered in this book, Riehl's model is unique in that it emphasises the capacity of people to give meaning to the events and situations they encounter and their interactions with others. *Meaning-giving*, as this process is known, is what leads two people to see the same situation in perhaps very different ways. Nurses, for example, may have little fear of the hospital environment in which they work. To them, the layout, the business, the noises and the smells of the hospital are familiar and are interpreted as such. To others who have less experience of this environment, however, hospitals can be very frightening places. Their endless corridors and staircases can lead many people to feel that they will get lost (or may never escape), and their smells and noises can cause people to fear the worst about the procedures that may be carried out within their walls.

This emphasis on people as givers of meaning to the events and situations they encounter is at one with the approach to explaining human behaviour developed by a group of social scientists called the social interactionists (Blumer, 1969). One of their most important members, Mead (1934), believed that a key human quality is the capacity to understand and relate to the world in terms of symbols. By the word 'symbol', he meant a word, image or action that stands for something else. We spend a lot of our time communicating with each other by way of symbols (smiles, nods, words, our style of dress, and so on). Hence, the term 'symbolic interactionist' is used to describe someone who finds this way of understanding individuals useful.

According to the symbolic interactionists, when people encounter unfamiliar situations, they try to make sense of them using their past experience, or the *stock of knowledge* that they have. Thus, meanings of events, objects, places and actions are not given but are actively created through processes of *interpretation*. Thomas (1967), another symbolic interactionist writer, believed that situations defined as real by people can become real in their consequences. For example, if a person feels that the environment he is in restricts his freedom and dignity, he may learn to become helpless within it. Alternatively, if he decides that it is supportive and likely to aid a speedy recovery from illness, it is all the more likely that such a recovery will take place.

All this could be taken to imply that the social world exists only in the eye of the beholder and that all that a person has to do to make something come true is to believe that it will do so. This is, of course, not true. Some interpretations of the world are more accurate than others, and any interpretation is open to challenge by others. People's definitions of reality and the symbolic universes they inhabit can and do change. The processes of communication and *negotiation* that take place between nurses and those for whom they care, lead to changes in perception and interpretation on both the nurse's and the client's part. This is central both to the process of care and to the process of either accepting a condition or becoming better.

One final element of symbolic interactionist thought central to Riehl's model is the notion of *role-taking*. By this is meant the capacity of individuals cognitively to internalise another person's perception of reality. Through role-taking, the nurse and the person for whom she is providing care, come closer together. She begins to understand better the way in which he sees the world as he begins to understand things better from the nurse's perspective. We develop a sense of self (our self-concept) by observing the reactions of others towards us, in other words, by role-taking. The *sick role* may be taken when we perceive ourselves to be ill, through the responses of others towards us or through other forms of symbolic interaction.

Key components of care

The nature of people

It follows from what has been said that people are first and foremost meaning-givers stimulated to act by the symbols that surround them. Beyond this, however, people differ in the manner in which they make sense of their circumstances and the events around them. In order to plan meaningful interventions with the individual, the nurse needs to develop insight into the way in which that person sees the world and his own status within it – as 'ill', as 'well', as in need of nursing care, for example. She will do this by taking the role of the other and trying to see the world through their eyes (Riehl, 1980; Riehl-Sisca, 1989). At the same time, the 'other' will be encouraged to understand things on the nurse's own terms. The ultimate goal of nursing is to guide the individual in:

maintaining and regaining a higher level of wellness to improve the quality of life and to gain insight during life's journey regardless of the health problem. (Riehl-Sisca, 1998)

The causes of problems likely to require intervention

According to Riehl-Sisca, nursing problems arise from disturbances within one or more of three *parameters* – physiological, psychological and sociological – affecting the individual's behaviour (Riehl-Sisca, 1989). Disturbance within any one of these may have consequences not only for that parameter, but for others as well. For example, psychological stresses brought on by being in a strange environment or being subject to competing expectations may have physiological consequences, while sociological factors, such as a change in job or daily routine, may have been responsible for these psychological stresses in the first place. That said, it is disturbances within the psychological and sociological parameters that are most likely to cause the kinds of problem requiring nursing support and intervention.

The nature of assessment

While Riehl-Sisca does not use the term 'assessment' extensively in her own writing, she emphasises the need to look carefully and systematically at various aspects of the person in making a judgement about his needs. In her early writing, Riehl-Sisca advocated the use of the FANCAP system of assessment developed by Abbey (1980) (Figure 12.1). FANCAP is a mnemonic that nurses can use to conduct an assessment of six areas of human activity. The attention that Riehl's model directs towards assessing the subjective dimensions of an individual's experience should, however, be noted.

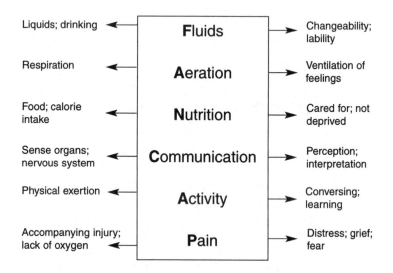

Liquids; drinking	**Fluids**	Changeability; lability
Respiration	**Aeration**	Ventilation of feelings
Food; calorie intake	**Nutrition**	Cared for; not deprived
Sense organs; nervous system	**Communication**	Perception; interpretation
Physical exertion	**Activity**	Conversing; learning
Accompanying injury; lack of oxygen	**Pain**	Distress; grief; fear

Figure 12.1   FANCAP – a system for the assessment of patient and client needs. Nurses assess each of the six aspects of patients specified by the mnemonic FANCAP, paying particular attention to the range of functions covered by each of these

It has more recently been suggested that a modified version of the FANCAP system of assessment, whereby the nurse identifies in turn the physiological, psychological, sociological, cultural and environmental factors associated with each area of human activity in which there is an identified problem, may be most suitable for undertaking an initial assessment (Hissa, 1998) (Figure 12.2).

	Physiological	Psychological	Sociological	Cultural	Environmental
Fluids					
Aeration					
Nutrition					
Communication					
Activity					
Pain					

Figure 12.2 Riehl interaction model assessment tool (after Hissa, 1998)

Regardless of the framework adopted, the nurse aims, at each point in assessment, to develop her insight into the individual's subjective perceptions of the problems affecting him. Subsequently, she may attempt with the person to identify the roles that have been adopted in the past when coping with each of these problems. Finally, she will want to know about the degree of role flexibility an individual has, in order to be able to anticipate potential problems later when encouraging the individual to take on new roles.

It is important to emphasise that role-taking will commence during the process of assessment as efforts are made by both nurse and client to understand events from each other's point of view.

The nature of planning and goal setting

Using the means at her disposal, the nurse then proceeds to negotiate a series of therapeutic goals. Information will be actively exchanged between the nurse and the person for whom she is caring, and mutual role-taking will be consolidated. A range of different types of knowledge is likely to be brought into the planning and goal-setting process by the nurse. It may include that derived from Rogerian theory, transactional analysis, psychoanalytic theory, sociological theory, crisis theory and reinforcement theory (Preisner, 1980).

The initial emphasis in planning is likely to be on setting short-term goals. These will allow the nurse to remain sensitive to the individual's changing needs and will allow her to revise her judgement as the relationship develops. Nursing goals should be actively negotiated between the nurse and the person receiving care for each of the problem areas identified during assessment. They should, of course, be recorded in patient-centred terms.

The focus of intervention during implementation of the care plan

The emphasis in intervention will be on the development of role flexibility to allow the person to respond more positively to the health constraints that he or she is facing. It may be necessary for the individual to take on a range of new roles depending on the nature and severity of the problems being faced. Some roles may be linked to the environment in which care is being provided (the hospital, for example), whereas others may relate more closely to the condition.

Further role-taking involving the client and the nurse will help the individual come to understand some of the new role options that are available. Role-taking is a crucial aspect of intervention since it encourages individuals to understand their present situation in different ways and, by taking on the role of others, helps them to prepare for new kinds of more beneficial social interaction.

Through role-taking, the nurse too benefits. She will, for example, be able to modify her own contribution to care by appreciating more fully the interpretations and position of the other. Riehl-Sisca talks also of the need for *interpretation* in this process and the value of making what she describes as *process recordings* as part of the intervention itself. By reviewing these process recordings, both client and nurse will be able to chart changes in perceptions and role performances.

The nature of evaluation

For nurses using this model of nursing, evaluation is likely to involve examining the extent to which individuals have acquired or developed new roles enabling them to cope more adequately with the problems identified. Evaluation in Riehl's model is not likely to be a one-off event that takes place after intervention. Instead, it is likely to be a part of the process of constant reassessment allowed for by role-taking between the individual and the nurse.

The role of the nurse

Riehl's model advocates that nurses should strive to involve themselves *inter-subjectively* in the world of the client. They should try to understand the meanings given to their experience by the people for whom they are providing care. Only by doing this will the nurse be able to make an accurate assessment of needs, and only by acting in this way will she be able to intervene therapeutically in order to help individuals to extend their role repertoires to cope with health-related stresses and demands.

Given the emphasis that Riehl's model places on role-taking as a mode of nursing intervention, the role of the nurse should be seen as *complementary* to that of the person who is receiving care. Nurses working with this particular model should aim to develop their skills of empathy and their capacity to work within a framework of trust and equality.

Using Riehl's model

To illustrate the use of Riehl's model in nursing practice, two examples will be considered. The first will look at the model's applicability in community psychiatric nursing with a male patient who has made a suicide attempt. The second will examine the model's use in an accident and emergency (A&E) department where a young girl drug user presents with infected injection sites. This second example deliberately focuses on a physical problem to show the suitability of Riehl's model to a wide range of circumstances.

To implement her model Riehl-Sisca suggests that nurses should carry out an assessment, make a nursing diagnosis, plan and carry out care. Thus, a traditional nursing process approach is advocated. In her writing about the model, Riehl-Sisca pays greatest attention to the process of assessment. This is often seen in the early stages of model development as it is in its scope for a comprehensive and reliable assessment that a model's utility begins to be evaluated.

Riehl-Sisca sees the process of implementing the Riehl inter-action model beginning when a problem is encountered. This is then followed by *much discussion* (Riehl-Sisca, 1989) so that the correct nursing diagnosis is made. She describes the implementation of action to meet goals continuing until an obstacle is reached, when further assessment will be required. This is similar to the continuous assessment seen as being appropriate to the model's philosophy of developing a relationship between patient and nurse (Aggleton and Chalmers, 1989).

The applicability of the Riehl interaction model in health promotion and health education needs to be considered carefully since an approach that is initiated by the identification of an actual problem may seem less than satisfactory. However,

Knauth and Gross (1989) have described the model's use in identifying and responding to the needs, rather than the problems, of
pregnant women and their families.

Assessment

Riehl-Sisca (1989: 394) favours an assessment matrix, illustrated
in Figure 12.2 above, based on five parameters detailed on the
horizontal plane and on the mnemonic FANCAP elaborated
vertically. The use of both the mnemonic device and the five
parameters as guides to assessment encourages attention not
only to the individuals' physical aspects, but also their psychological and social concerns. Such attention should produce high-
quality data on which to plan the delivery of nursing care.
Knauth and Gross (1989) have described a modified assessment
matrix that includes a Likert scale leading to a numerical score.
Despite the fact that this features in Riehl-Sisca's (1989) edited
text *Conceptual Models for Nursing Practice*, it seems to fit uneasily
with the underlying commitments of the model and as such will
not be used here.

Nurses working with the Riehl model should not be
prescriptive about what they believe the patient's problem to
be. Riehl-Sisca (1989: 399) puts this powerfully when identifying strategies for implementing her model: 'Listen to the
patient, family, accept, believe and trust them to know what is
best for them.' Rather than being prescriptive, nurses should
take time to understand the meaning of what is happening to
the patient. Unusual or potentially harmful behaviours will
pose special challenges for nurses trying to access patients'
reasons for their actions.

This is shown in the first example, where a community
psychiatric nurse is beginning to form a therapeutic relationship
with a man who has made an attempt on his own life. Her first
encounter with the patient may be in an acute, medical inpatient
setting prior to the man's discharge after a suicide attempt. This
may be a brief meeting in preparation for the offer of further help
in the man's home, the main assessment taking place over the
next few days.

In keeping with the concerns of symbolic interactionist theory,
the nurse will use the assessment matrix to help her gather information to aid her understanding of the symbols, meanings and

values operating in the man's world and influencing his actions. To achieve this, the nurse may engage in role-taking to enhance her insight into the patient's perspective.

She may discover, for example, that the man feels that his future is bleak. He may be facing redundancy, feel that without work his life will lack purpose and think that his chances of getting another job are remote. He may have worries about his financial security and about the loss of the companionship offered by his work colleagues. The nurse may tentatively identify several problems. The first may be in relation to loss of his normal work (activity) within the psychological parameter. Not working may mean that he sees himself having fewer opportunities for personal growth and development.

There may also be problems of distress and fear (pain) about the potential loss of companionship linked to the environmental parameter. In addition, the nurse may, in trying to understand why he attempted to commit suicide, wonder whether there is a difficulty to do with talking to someone else about how he is feeling (aeration). She may regard this as originating within the cultural parameter, adult men traditionally feeling it inappropriate to discuss personal problems with others. To remain consistent with the model's ideals, the nurse will need to validate with the man what she believes are his problems. Only when these have been confirmed will it be reasonable to begin the planning process.

The nurse working in an A&E department may find herself trying to assist a young girl who injects herself with illegal substances and who is worried because some of her injection sites are red and sore. Whatever the nurse's feelings about injecting drug use, she must remain sensitive to the importance of the activity for the girl. Primarily, her role is to help with what the girl perceives to be her problem, in this case areas of skin infection. The success of her intervention with regard to this problem may or may not lead to other opportunities to offer help. It may also be that the girl immediately becomes uncomfortable in a hospital environment where various symbols such as notices to patients and uniforms indicate a place where control rests largely with the staff.

The nurse will want to find out the extent of the physical problem by examining all the sites that the girl uses. This will help determine the degree of injury (pain), in the physiological parameter, to the skin and underlying tissues. She will also encourage the girl to explain her injection technique in detail, including her understanding of the need for the equipment to be initially sterile and used only once, and for the procedure to be clean. It may be that the girl has a gap in her understanding, in the psychological parameter (communication), about the careful use of sterile equipment so that it is still clean when entering the skin. This might be exacerbated by the girl's living conditions where she is deprived (nutrition) of ready access to washing facilities. The nurse may identify this as a problem within the environmental parameter.

For the nurse to gather data about the girl's lifestyle and living conditions demands considerable trust on the girl's behalf, especially if she feels uneasy in the hospital setting. It may be that only the physical problem can be addressed if she is unwilling to give information about anything else. The nurse working with the Riehl-Sisca model should not feel that she has failed in her assessment if only limited information is forthcoming. The nurse–patient relationship hinges on the meaning of the situation for the patient, and if the girl only wants her skin problem to be addressed, the nurse must accept this. She can briefly explain that there are other ways in which she might be able to help, but it is the girl's right to proceed or otherwise.

Planning

As the nurse–patient relationship develops, the nurse will gain a greater understanding of the patient's perceptions of his or her problems. Also, as the care episode evolves, the patient's perceptions themselves may change. For these reasons, jointly negotiated, short-term goals are likely to be the most useful in implementing the Riehl interaction model as they allow for sensitive and timely adjustments to what is planned. Riehl-Sisca (1989) has also advocated making use, if possible, of any past coping mechanisms identified during assessment.

The man who attempted suicide may see death as the best way out of his current difficulties. The nurse working with this model will want to do all she can to help him to find alternative strategies to cope with his problems. More traditional medicalised approaches to care might find nurses engaged in round-the-clock supervision in order to stop any suicide attempts. With the Riehl model, this would rarely be part of the plan of care unless the patient himself requested it. Working with this model means that all measures reasonable and acceptable to the patient should be used to preserve life, but ultimately the patient has the right to choose. Riehl-Sisca (1989: 399) makes it clear that once patients have been informed of pertinent and up-to-date knowledge and have been given the opportunity to discuss alternatives, 'it is their choice, it is their life'.

The community psychiatric nurse will therefore initially want to negotiate a short-term goal of allowing time for her to tell the man what she can offer in the way of help and what alternative coping strategies there are other than suicide. If this is achieved, the opportunity is there for further short-term goals to be set. A probable sequence of goals might be to address next the problem to do with aeration so that the man can gain some personal support from somebody else. In the short term, this might be the nurse herself, but another goal will be to select a suitable friend or relative whom the man feels could offer him help.

The problems related to pain and activity may then be thought about and possibly some tentative plans made. However, for someone whose despondency has been marked enough for him to attempt suicide, it is likely that these other problems will remain unaddressed for some considerable time. For the planning of his care to remain meaningful for the man, any suggestion that such difficulties are high on his agenda for action is liable to be dismissed as irrelevant. The understandings on which the Riehl model is based offer positive reasons why known problems may need to be ignored in the short term. Everything in the care episode must be meaningful and acceptable to the patient. Also, using short-term goals in preference to long-term ones allows for adjustments to what is planned as and when this seems appropriate.

For the girl in the A&E department, the short-term goal of priority might be to reduce the pain and soreness around the injection sites. To this end, she and the nurse may negotiate a daily meeting for several days for local treatment to the sites. The nurse will also want to identify any organisms in the wounds that might be sensitive to antibiotic therapy. She may therefore seek the girl's agreement for interventions designed to identify any offending organisms and for the possible involvement in her care of an A&E doctor who can prescribe appropriate medication.

The nurse's knowledge of the potential risks of such infections in an injecting drug user may mean that she also wants to plan for further checks on the girl's current health status. She may seek agreement for other tests such as a daily body temperature recording and a full blood count.

As the relationship between the girl and the nurse develops, it may be possible to establish goals in relation to the girl's under-standing, or communication problem, about injection technique and about her lack of nurturing in the environment in which she lives. For example, the nurse might ask whether the girl would be willing to demonstrate the technique she uses so that the nurse can gain a greater understanding of its strengths and weaknesses. They might then agree a longer-term goal to improve the girl's understanding of asepsis and its relevance to her particular lifestyle and health.

With regard to living conditions, the nurse might negotiate with the girl a plan to return to this aspect once the main goal of reducing the pain and soreness the girl is experiencing has been met. While the girl is in pain and possibly feeling unwell as a result of infection, it would be unlikely that she would see her own living conditions as a high priority. By accepting that goals in this area need to be addressed at a later date, the nurse is demonstrating sensitivity to the girl's situation in a way that reflects the concerns of this particular model.

Implementation of action

Riehl-Sisca (1989) argues that there is a relationship between the concepts of communication, self and role. Most importantly, she uses role theory to help to explain lowered self-concept and a decrease in communication. She believes that individuals can take on a number of roles and that it is when few roles are taken on that a person's self-esteem and confidence are threatened. This is exemplified by the man facing redundancy who will therefore lose important roles as an employee and an earner. With this model, therefore, nursing aims to assist patients to develop greater role flexibility so that they can cope better with health-related demands.

Riehl-Sisca identifies a number of roles that nurses themselves might utilise during the implementation stage, including those of problem-solver, teacher, change agent and role model to the patient. In each case, a reciprocal role is required from the patient. In these examples, the patient's role would be a seeker of a problem solution, a learner, a change agent novice, and an observer and doer.

For the man who attempted suicide, the nurse may hope to teach him to extend his repertoire of roles such that he can develop other strategies to cope with his problems. Assuming that he is prepared to discuss what she has to offer, the nurse may first want to encourage him to talk about what is happening to him and how he is feeling. For him to see value and meaning in this, she may ask him to tell her about other occasions in his life when he has been helped by talking to someone. Alternatively, he may be able to relate a time when he helped someone else by listening to concerns and offering support. The nurse may encourage him to role-take (think about a situation from another's point of view) the position of someone he cares for who might be in distress and seeking help.

By encouraging him in role-taking, the nurse might help him to achieve a greater intersubjective understanding about his current difficulties. In addition, he may begin to see alternative meanings and alternative roles for himself in the present situation. He might begin to understand that people who care for each other wish to help even in what appears to be a desperate situation. In this way, he might start to see possible benefits in ventilating his feelings and fears to someone he trusts. By offering him time and encouragement, the nurse will be acting as the role model of a good listener and supporter.

Riehl-Sisca also sees the nurse as someone who can encourage the patient to accept care from others. During the implementation stage, therefore, the nurse will be hoping to help the man to identify other people among his friends and family who will be able to provide him with ongoing support. If he moves beyond wanting to commit suicide, the man may acknowledge that his ability to come to terms with his changed prospects depends on his accepting continuing help from both the nurse and selected others who care for him and with whom he can communicate openly.

The main goal for the girl attending the A&E department is to have less discomfort from her injection sites, which had become infected. To this end, the nurse will clean any open sores and apply appropriate dressings where needed. If the girl seems responsive to the idea, the nurse may talk through the nursing technique for carrying out a dressing as she does it. In this way, she may be able to help the girl's understanding of the principles involved in trying to avoid infection. The use of pain-relieving tablets may also have a place in the girl's care in the short term.

The nurse will take wound swabs from various injection sites so that any antibiotic treatment can occur in response to identi-fied organisms and sensitivities (problem-solving). With the girl's permission, she may take and record her body temperature at each visit to check for signs of systemic infection. Depending on the extent of the infection and on the symptoms displayed, it may be necessary to involve medical staff in the girl's care if she agrees. This could be to prescribe antibiotic therapy and to take blood samples.

In order for nursing actions to take place, the nurse will need to ensure that everything possible is done to make re-attendance at the A&E department acceptable to the patient. She might therefore make an appointment time that means she herself will be available to provide continuity of care. Much of the success of the Riehl interaction model depends on the development of a meaningful relationship between patient and nurse. This is not possible if the patient sees a different nurse at each visit.

The nurse will also want to ascertain what it is about the department that makes the girl feel ill at ease. Some things (for example permanent notices), she will not be able to alter but in keeping with the commitments of the model, she may be able to extend the girl's understanding of the meaning of, and need for, some of these symbols. She might, for example, encourage her to role-take being a nurse in an A&E department so that she might regard the wearing of uniforms somewhat differently. Time spent in such activities, with the nurse in the role as change agent, may go some way towards helping the girl attend regularly for nursing care.

If the relationship develops into one of increasing trust, the nurse may later be able to adopt the role of teacher in an effort better to address the goals related to communication and nurtu-rance. The girl may agree to demonstrate her injection tech-nique so that safe aspects can be identified and positively reinforced, and weaker elements altered to make them safer. Together, the nurse and the girl may discuss strategies to ensure that greater opportunities are created for the girl to keep her skin clean.

Evaluation

As with the majority of models, the Riehl-Sisca model is initially evaluated by reference to the meeting or otherwise of goals set at the planning stage of the nursing process. Very often, this will incorporate examining the extent to which patients have developed role flexibility and new role performances. Observable patient behaviour will therefore be important in judging goal achievement, as will be the patient's opinion about the role(s) he or she feels able to take on.

The man who attempted suicide was initially encouraged to allow the nurse time to offer him help through discussion. If this is achieved, a short-term goal will be set to enable him to talk about his problems with another person. His success in developing this new role might be evaluated in terms of the amount of time he is willing to spend discussing his difficulties with the nurse and the content of the discussion. The implementation of the Riehl model might be deemed successful if he is able to discuss his feelings in some depth.

Later evaluation might focus on the development of a similar relationship with a member of his family or with a friend. Any positive outcome in meeting these early short-term goals might be judged even more favourably if the man is ultimately able to move on to plan goals in relation to the problems of pain (distress and fear) and activity (loss of normal work).

For the young girl with infected injection sites, formative evaluation will also initially focus on her willingness to accept help from the nurse and to reattend the A&E department as planned. While goals such as these do not effect a direct change related to the health difficulty, in this case the infected sites, they are extremely important in enabling people to take on a role that enables them to access appropriate health care. There is evidence to suggest that, in this as in other areas of nursing practice, those most in need of care are often the most reluctant to access it.

If the girl attends for treatment, the goals related to relieving her pain and discomfort can be evaluated at each visit. In part, the nurse will want to see physical signs of wound healing and a decrease in inflammation and exudate, but she will very importantly also want to know whether the girl feels less discomfort. A pain chart could be a useful tool here, along with a careful record of the healing progress of each site. This could include written descriptions, diagrams or even photographs if the girl agrees to this.

In the longer term, evaluation may consider how willing the girl is to have help in improving her injection technique, and ultimately the absence of soreness and infection around her injection sites. The latter is extremely difficult to evaluate as non-attendance may be difficult to interpret. It may mean that the patient has no further problems, but does not necessarily indicate that this is the case.

Nurses working with this model will also want to evaluate its usefulness summatively. This can only take place when the model has been used and carefully evaluated with a number of different people with a range of health care problems. What may be discovered is that the Riehl model, like other models, has particular strengths when used in particular fields. First, the acknowledgement that all behaviour is meaningful should act as a spur to nurses concerned with the difficulties often encountered in reaching those people most in need of health care but who seem unwilling to access care opportunities. This model encourages nurses to seek to understand the signs and symbols that might be acting as barriers to the use of health care services for those at risk or in need.

Second, it highlights the importance of continuity of care for people seeking health advice or health care. The success of this model rests heavily on the developing relationship between patient and nurse. This becomes difficult, if not impossible, in a care environment where nurses are constantly changing and cannot offer a commitment to a continuing relationship. The model's use will be significantly more successful where nurses have negotiated greater autonomy and can organise their work in the patients' best interests. In theory, the introduction of named nurses should facilitate the growth of relationships in health care that maximise the potential of models such as that of Riehl. The reality is, however, that reducing numbers of trained nurses is likely to have an impact on the success of all interactionist models.

References

Abbey, J. (1980) FANCAP: What is it? In Riehl, J.P. and Roy, C. (eds) *Conceptual Models for Nursing Practice*, 2nd edn. Norwalk, CT, Appleton-Century-Crofts.

Aggleton, P.J. and Chalmers, H.A. (1989) Working with the Riehl model of nursing. In Riehl-Sisca J.P. (ed.) *Conceptual Models for Nursing Practice*, 3rd edn. Norwalk, CT, Appleton and Lange.

Blumer, H. (1969) *Symbolic Interactionism: Perspective and Method*. Englewood Cliffs, NJ, Prentice-Hall.

Hissa, D. (1998) Riehl-Sisca interaction model assessment tool. In Tomey, A.M. and Alligood, M.R. (eds) *Nursing Theorists and their Work*, 4th edn. St Louis, C.V. Mosby.

Knauth, D.G. and Gross, E.B. (1989) The Riehl interaction model prenatal family assessment tool for the childbirth educator. In Riehl-Sisca, J.P. (ed.) *Conceptual Models for Nursing Practice*, 3rd edn. Norwalk, CT, Appleton & Lange.

Mead, G.H. (1934) *Mind, Self and Society*. Chicago, University of Chicago Press.

Preisner, J.M. (1980) A proposed model for the nurse therapist. In Riehl, J.P. and Roy, C. (eds) *Conceptual Models for Nursing Practice*, 2nd edn. Norwalk, CT, Appleton-Century-Crofts.

Riehl, J.P. (1980) The Riehl interaction model. In Riehl, J.P. and Roy, C. (eds) *Conceptual Models for Nursing Practice*, 2nd edn. Norwalk, CT, Appleton-Century-Crofts.

Riehl-Sisca, J.P. (1989) The Riehl interaction model. In Riehl-Sisca, J.P. (ed.) *Conceptual Models for Nursing Practice*, 3rd edn. Norwalk, CT, Appleton & Lange.

Riehl-Sisca, J.P. (1998) Personal correspondence. Cited in Tomey, A.M. and Alligood, M.R. *Nursing Theorists and their Work*, 4th edn. St Louis, C.V. Mosby.

Thomas, W.I. (1967) *The Unadjusted Girl*. New York, Harper & Row.

Chapter 13 Rogers' unitary field model of nursing

We will end our consideration of nursing models by examining a unique approach to the planning and delivery of care, and one of the most controversial – Rogers' unitary field model of nursing. Martha Rogers trained as a nurse at Knoxville General Hospital School of Nursing in the 1930s. After working in rural nursing in Michigan, she became a visiting nurse supervisor and educator first in Connecticut and later in Phoenix, Arizona. She completed her graduate study at Teachers College, Columbia University and Johns Hopkins University in Baltimore. For over 20 years, she was Professor and Head of the Division of Nursing at New York University. She died in 1994, recognised as one of the most 'stimulating, challenging, controversial, idealistic, visionary, prophetic, philosophic, academic, outspoken, humorous, blunt and ethical' (Tomey and Alligood, 1998: 208) nurse scholars there have been.

In contrast to the majority of nursing models we have looked at, that of Rogers is more abstract in nature. By blending together insights from a wide range of disciplines, including astronomy, physics, biology, psychology, sociology and anthropology, Rogers suggests that humans are best understood not as systems or discrete parts, but as unified fields of energy that interact with their environments (Rogers, 1970, 1983, 1992). Such a view shares some features in common with traditional beliefs about health and the systems of health care that preceded modern medicine. Among native peoples in North America, throughout much of Asia even today and in the Mediterranean world until the late sixteenth century, approaches to health care emphasised *holism* and the irreducibility of people to their bodily systems and parts.

According to such perspectives, physical and psychological conditions as varied as weakness, dizziness, confusion, fainting and many other health-related complaints are said to result from problems of energy imbalance. In traditional Chinese medicine, for example, imbalances in the flow of life energy (Ch'i) lead to physical and psychological illness and may be caused by an imbalance between the individual's body rhythms and those to be found outside the person in nature. Lunar and solar cycles, as well as meteorological and climatic conditions, establish energy systems that interact with those of the person. It is the simultaneous rhythmical interaction between these systems that determines an individual's state of well-being. Health care intervention focuses holistically upon the person in an attempt to restore the free flow of energy throughout the body and soul. Massage, acupuncture, moxybustion (applying the burning ash of the mugwort plant to energy points in the body) and herbal remedies have an important role to play in allowing this to happen (Krieger, 1981).

Among ayurvedic health practitioners in the Indian subcontinent and elsewhere, health-related interventions are also holistic in nature. Here, efforts are made to restore the balance between three primary bodily humours: vata (wind), pitha (gall) and kapha (mucus). Following an examination of the quality of different pulses, the ayurvedic practitioner may intervene by suggesting naturopathic remedies, changes in diet and exercise, and perhaps the use of yoga to re-establish the balance between the individual and the broader universe of which he or she is a part. Interestingly, similar ideas informed the European holistic approach to health care favoured by the ancient Greeks and by the followers of physician Galen. This emphasised the existence of four bodily humours: blood, mucus, yellow bile and black bile. Imbalances between these were again detected (among other means) through an examination of pulses, and intervention sought to restore the overall equilibrium between individuals and their environments.

A number of important themes run through each of the above approaches to health and health care. First, each of them shows *holism* in the sense that it emphasises the integrity of people and the foolishness of efforts to reduce them to constituent parts. Second, each draws attention to what might be described as *rhythmicity* or the idea that there are cycles or resonances between people and their environments. Third, each works with a notion of *potentiality*, which suggests there may be untapped sources of energy within the person that can be used for healing.

Until relatively recently, many of these ideas would have been unfamiliar to those working in health care. However, a growing interest in complementary medicine has focused attention on the value of more 'holistic' understandings of people and their needs. Curiosity with regard to the potential of practices as diverse as acupuncture and acupressure, hypnotherapy and meditation, chiropractic and osteopathy, to enhance health and well-being has led many nurses to experiment with these approaches as part of an overall approach to care. While Rogers (1983) has explicitly rejected the use of the term 'holistic' to describe her model, preferring the adjective 'unitary' instead, there are some similarities of emphasis and approach.

Key components of care

The nature of people

According to Rogers, it is a mistake to view people as individuals composed of physiological, psychological and social systems. Instead, human beings are best understood as dynamic *fields of energy*, which are themselves a part of broader environmental energy fields. The *unitary human field*, (as Rogers describes the person) is an:

irreducible, indivisible, pandimensional energy field identified by pattern and manifesting characteristics that are specific to the whole and that cannot be predicted from the parts. (Tomey and Alligood, 1998: 209).

The human energy field is integral to (that is a part of) the environmental energy field, and it is the potential synergy between these two fields (that is the capacity of one to influence the other beneficially) of which nurses should be aware when thinking about human problems and needs. When two or more individuals act in relationship to one another, a *group energy field* is likely to arise. Like unitary human fields, group energy fields are irreducible and indivisible.

According to Rogers, energy fields are open (that is subject to influence by other fields), infinite and integral to one another. She calls this idea the 'universe of open systems'. Human and environmental fields, as well as being integral to one another, are in a condition of constant interaction and change. Human energy fields display what Rogers calls *pattern*, or distinguishing characteristics. Pattern changes with time and while not directly observable, gives rise to *manifestations*: behaviours and qualities of that individual or unitary human field. The manifestations may include a sense of self or may appear in the form of ways of responding to the environment, such as by being fast or slow, or in the form of imaginative or pragmatic responses.

Energy fields show what Rogers calls 'pandimensionality'. Rogers finds the notion of a three-dimensional world unsatisfactory when it comes to explaining human beings. Her acceptance of aspects of the paranormal in the form of *déjà vu* and clairvoyance encourages her to understand human energy fields as being in interaction with others in ways and through dimensions that are not yet fully understood. Nurses should be sensitive to this possibility in their everyday practice.

Finally, Rogers identifies what she calls three 'principles of homeodynamics', which characterise the relationship between human and other energy fields. The first of these principles, that of *integrality* (called 'complementarity' in Rogers, 1980), highlights the constant interaction between the human energy field and environmental energy fields. The second principle – *helicy* – describes how human and environmental change occurs. Rogers suggests (somewhat optimistically perhaps) that this is usually in the direction of continuous innovation and increased complexity. Finally, the principle of *resonancy* describes the tendency for human energy fields to change so that higher-frequency wave patterns appear as time goes by. Both hyperactivity in children and the more frequent patterns of sleeping and awakening in the elderly are cited as examples of this general human tendency.

The causes of problems likely to require intervention

According to Rogers, the need for nursing care will arise when there is an imbalance between the unitary human energy field and the environmental energy field. Many factors can cause such an imbalance, including physical and physiological disturbance as well as psychological, social and environmental stress.

The nature of assessment – pattern appraisal

Rogers does not often use the terms 'assessment', 'planning' and 'goal-setting' in her writing. Instead, she talks of the need for the nurse to appraise the unitary energy field of the other, while recognising that both it and her own unitary field are integral to the environmental field. Cowling (1990) has developed a frequently used system for pattern appraisal in which efforts are made through observation and participation to access the perceptions, experience and reflections of the other as a unitary whole.

This kind of approach aims to go beyond systems of assessment that seek to reduce the complexity and wholeness of people to systems and constituent parts. It emphasises a process of mutual exploration as efforts are made better to understand the organisation of the individual's unitary energy field and its relationship with others. A range of techniques may be used in appraisal, including empathetic conversation, professional closeness and forms of therapeutic touch (Krieger, 1979).

As stated above, 'planning' and 'goal-setting' are not terms explicitly used in Rogers' framework. Instead, the emphasis is on the alleviation of *dis-ease*. That said, it is possible to imagine the setting of immediate and longer-term goals linking to the restoration of equilibrium in human energy systems and the facilitation of synergy between them and those of the environment.

The focus of intervention during implementation of the care plan – mutual patterning

While drugs and technological interventions have a useful role to play in alleviating some of the more immediate causes of disease, the long-term effectiveness of these approaches is to be doubted in the absence of concurrent attempts to restore balance within human energy fields. A range of interventions may be useful in doing this. These include meditation, guided imagery, guided reminiscence and memory work. Physical exercise, 'sleep hygiene' (Parker, 1989) and art and music therapy may also have an important role to play in reducing dis-ease. More physical kinds of intervention may include body massage and therapeutic touch as well as acupuncture and acupressure. Indeed, many of the kinds of intervention looked upon with some suspicion by modern biomedical practitioners find a place within the framework for nursing care that Rogers advocates. Regardless of the approach adopted, the emphasis remains on the unitary individual throughout nursing intervention, and on restoring equilibrium and synergy between their energy field and that of the immediate or potential environment.

The nature of evaluation

In her analysis of the use of Rogers model, Quinn (1981) acknowledges that assessing the extent to which an energy field has been successfully repatterned is unlikely to be a simple process. A number of factors may be looked for, however, as evidence of therapeutic success. These include a greater awareness on the part of the individual of the relationship between environmental factors and his or her problems. More subtle changes in energy balance and response may require empathetic and even intuitive assessment by the nurse throughout the constantly evolving process of mutual patterning.

The role of the nurse

According to Rogers (1970: 122), the major goal of nursing is to promote:

symphonic interaction between [people and their] environment, to strengthen the coherence and integrity of the human field, and to direct and re-direct patterning of the human and environmental fields for realisation of maximum human health potential.

The role of the nurse links closely to these ideas in that she must be sensitive to individual needs (while recognising that these link to wider environmental circumstances), able to recognise patterns and willing to accept the connectedness of events and processes. The uniqueness of the individual is central to Rogers' approach, this being a value that the nurse working with this model must hold. Beyond this, however, Rogerian nurses are likely to be skilled in the application of a wide range of social and bodily interventions including the use of guided imagery, therapeutic touch, music, exercise and art as forms of therapy.

Using Rogers' model

The challenges posed by Rogers' model may be viewed with scepticism by some health professionals, particularly those whose training and experience within health care have been heavily influenced by traditional, medicalised approaches to patients and their diseases. While a questioning and critical stance is to be welcomed when new ideas are being evaluated, there must be an accompanying willingness to see value and potential where it exists. Some mainstream health care provision is already recognising the contribution to patient well-being that can be gained by offering alternative approaches to traditional care. For example, it is now not unusual to find practitioners such as acupuncturists and homeopathists working in health centres alongside GPs and practice nurses.

What remains important is for the particular approach to the delivery of health care to be one that is acceptable to the patient and one that offers the chance of genuine benefit for the problem being experienced. Rogers' model might, therefore, not be the model of choice for someone who is looking for a traditional consultation focusing on a specific and limited local problem such as a sore throat. Equally, it might not be the right approach in an emergency situation when speedy intervention is required to preserve life. However, it may be a valuable model to use when trying to address complex problems of dis-ease that do not lend themselves to traditional, reductionist approaches to care.

The examples given in this chapter illustrate two such dilemmas. The first considers the difficulties faced by a young married couple whose son has not yet started school and who is thought to be overactive. The second focuses on the distress of an elderly woman with short-term memory loss who lives in a residential home.

Pattern appraisal

For a nurse working with Rogers' model, gaining an understanding about an individual or a family and their dis-ease is likely to be a process rather different from that encountered with other models. To begin with, human beings are, according to Rogers, energy fields that are unitary. In other words, people are not *made up* of energy fields, they *are* energy fields (Rogers, 1989) and are consequently not reducible to a number of parts. Appraisal will therefore always seek information and understanding about the whole person or the whole family, even though there may be a focus on particular manifestations. In addition, some of the methods used by a Rogerian nurse during the appraisal process may well seem unique to this model. As identified above, these may include empathetic conversations, professional closeness and forms of therapeutic touch.

Increasingly, the value of caring for children in their own homes is being recognised, and the overactive child described in this chapter might therefore be referred to a paediatric community nurse. As a Rogerian nurse, she would see him as a human energy field integral to the energy fields of his parents and his enviroment. From the time the nurse first visits the family, her own energy field also becomes integral to those of the child and his family. This marks the beginning of her professional closeness with them.

Gaining an understanding of the dynamic relationship between the child's energy field and those of his parents and his environment may take some time. It is likely that the nurse will want to talk with the child and the parents both together and separately (empathetic conversations) in an effort to integrate herself further into their energy fields. She will ask the parents to describe in detail the characteristic behaviours they perceive their son to manifest and which they regard as problematic. She will seek information about any variation in his behaviour over the course of a normal day and will want to know about his sleep patterns. She may discover that he goes to sleep much later than other children of his age, usually wakes about 5 am and then goes immediately to wake his parents.

If he is willing and able, she will talk with the little boy himself about how he likes to spend his time and about anything he dislikes doing. She will also want opportunities to observe the child at play and during other activities to make her own appraisal of the level of his activity and whether it is 'normal' for his age and developmental stage. With the parents' agreement, she may spend time alone with the boy to watch how he occupies himself with toys and other pastimes when his parents are not there.

The second example concerns an elderly woman recently admitted to a residential home, an environment in which many nurses now work and where many of the challenges posed differ considerably from those usually encountered in an acute hospital setting. The elderly woman may show signs of considerable disease, manifested particularly by repeated wandering around the home and verbal expressions of anxiety.

The focus of pattern appraisal will be in trying to find out about the lack of harmony between the woman's energy field and that of her immediate environment, particularly as she is having to adjust to new and strange surroundings. The nurse will initially want to establish some professional closeness with the woman in order to gain her trust. This will be made more difficult by the woman's short-term memory loss as she may at first repeatedly forget who the nurse is.

During appraisal, the nurse may discover that the woman's short-term memory loss is so great that she feels permanently lonely and that this makes her feel very vulnerable and frightened. Despite time spent with her by both nurses and visitors, she may, once they leave her, forget straight away that they have ever been there. She may peceive her days to be endless and boring. Her own solution to this is to walk around the home environment seeking people out and displaying restlessness as a manifestation of her dis-ease.

Conversations with the woman may reveal that she looks more relaxed and is prepared to sit in one place for a period of time when she is encouraged to talk about her past. She may have a store of memories, the recounting of which show her in a very different light and help to inform the nurse about how her previous life has been conducted. The nurse may also ask friends and relatives for more information to help her get an image of what life was like for the woman when she was more in harmony with her environment. She may discover that, in particular, the routines of the home and the kinds of activity in which most of the residents take part are largely alien to the elderly woman she is appraising.

She may find out that the woman had been very successful in business and had owned several high-class shops. On retirement, her skills turned to making her home beautiful, and much of her day had been spent doing household chores and in having friends in for coffee or tea. She had rarely watched television, read fictional texts or played games, all common activities in many residential homes.

Throughout the appraisal process, the nurse will be continuously processing the information she gains. For the paediatric community nurse, this processing may be informed by her knowledge of other children and their families, and by her theoretical knowledge of child development. For the nurse working with elderly people, she will take into account both her knowledge of how older people behave when their short-term memory is impaired and her knowledge of the ageing process. Where the

Rogerian nurse may differ from nurses working with other models is that she will also come to the appraisal process with a knowledge gained from Rogers' understanding of the nature of people. Rogers has argued that the principles of homeodynamics support the theory of accelerating evolution (Rogers, 1989) and that this puts a different perspective on children's behaviour and people's longer waking periods. She also describes alterations in time perception for older people that have yet to be fully explored in relation to memory loss.

At all stages of the appraisal process, a nurse working with Rogers' model will want to ensure that the individual, whether a child or an adult, is participating in an informed manner in what is taking place. Appraisal can be seen as the first step in a process of change, and Rogers advocates that such a process should be undertaken *knowingly*.

Partnership in goal-setting

As indicated earlier in this chapter, Rogers has little to say about goal-setting. Mills and Biley (1994) argue that a traditional approach to nursing practice (in which goal-setting might be a part) is not to be found in the science of unitary human beings. Instead, they see Rogers' work as having the potential to guide nursing away from traditional approaches and towards something more creative. In view of the non-prescriptive nature of care with a Rogerian philosophy, the notion of a *partnership* (also used by Mills and Biley) for deciding the way forward seems appropriate.

The aim of nursing with Rogers' model is to help people to achieve maximum well-being within their potential. This is done by harmonising their energy field with those of their environment and of other individuals contributing to that environment.

For the paediatric community nurse working with the over-active boy and his family, the first issue to be addressed following pattern appraisal might be a greater exploration of the nature of the problem. In other words, she might feel that some goals can be realistically set in relation to the boy's activity level but that, overall, much of the difficulty rests with his parents' expectations of what constitutes 'normal' behaviour.

In negotiation with the boy and his parents, therefore, the nurse might suggest two rather different but parallel sets of goals. On the one hand, there may be goals to modify the child's behaviour, but in addition, there may be goals related to the parents' understanding of the variety of levels of activity seen in young children. For example, goals might be set in relation to the little boy going to sleep earlier and in relation to the time at which he wakes his parents in the morning. A goal for them could be to feel more accepting of his unique behaviour by gaining a greater understanding of it.

Goal-setting for the woman with short-term memory loss will pose particular challenges because she will probably not be able to participate in a partnership to determine the goals of care, and the potential to repattern her energy field may be limited. However, she may be able to identify that she dislikes feeling anxious and does not feel at ease with her new environment. For the nurse, this may be a sufficient starting point for planning interventions. The nurse may tentatively decide that changes are needed to better integrate the woman's energy field with that of the home environment, and that an attempt should be made to reproduce the woman's home environment as far as is possible. In this way, she would hope to replace restlessness with patterns of peace (Lutjens, 1991).

Mutual patterning

As we have seen, Rogers' model of nursing offers a framework within which what are currently regarded as innovative and creative approaches to nursing intervention are seen as entirely appropriate. Thus, the Rogerian nurse will be open to a consideration of a variety of approaches to care that come into the broad category of 'holistic' interventions (despite Rogers' dislike of the popular usage of the term 'holistic'). Methods will include techniques such as therapeutic touch, guided imagery, acupuncture, music therapy and aromatherapy, and nurses working with this model will therefore want to develop knowledge and skills in these and related areas.

Helping a child to modify his behaviour is particularly challenging when the child himself is unlikely to perceive any problem with what he does and when most interventions will ideally be carried out by his parents with teaching and support from the paediatric community nurse. Following careful appraisal, the nurse may be aware that certain manifestations in the child's environment seem to increase or decrease his activity level. These might include background noise, lighting and the response of others to his behaviour. She may have observed that he responds well to loving physical contact. She will aim to intervene to effect change in his own energy field and his environmental energy field.

The nurse may introduce his parents to the potential benefits of therapeutic touch or body massage. Sayre-Adams (1995) regards therapeutic touch as a useful therapy for insomnia, and the boy's parents might be encouraged to develop skills in the technique themselves. Many authors (for example Longworth, 1982; Balke *et al.*, 1989; Horrigan, 1995) have written of the benefits of body massage, with therapeutic gain in areas such as stress and muscle tension relief. It might also be a useful intervention for the little boy at bedtime and involves skills that his parents could learn.

To achieve a change in his behaviour on first waking, the nurse may suggest that certain play items, ones that he can manage safely and alone, are available in his bedroom. If he is able to tell the time, she may seek his agreement on a time before which he does not disturb his parents. She may also suggest that quiet music is tried as a way of helping him to behave in a calmer manner. A longer-term intervention might involve decorating his room in quiet colours and providing curtains that reduce the morning light. Atherton (1995) has also recommended the use of belladonna and agaricus for what he terms 'hyperactive children'.

The boy's parents may be helped by learning more about variations in children's behaviour and particularly by being introduced to Rogers' ideas about accelerating evolution as a theory developed from the principles of homeodynamics. In this, she argues that many pathological labels, hyperactivity in children being one such term, fail to recognise that new norms have been generated over time by higher-frequency wave patterns (resonancy). In particular, Rogers argues that 'gifted children and the so-called hyperactive' may show increased waking periods and more diverse sleep patterns (Rogers, 1989: 186). The nurse may provide relevant literature for the parents to read, with an opportunity to then discuss with her what they have read.

For the elderly woman, the nurse is hoping to establish greater harmony between her energy field and that of the residential home environment. In many such homes, residents bring with them some of their own furniture and possessions, but the nurse may liaise with the woman's relatives for more of her own things to be brought to her. She may encourage the woman to re-engage in familiar activities such as household chores. Thus, she may carry out some cleaning in her own room and may help the domestic staff employed in the home. This will have the added benefit of providing opportunities for being with people so that she feels less alone.

Guided reminiscence and memory work may also be interventions of value. Drawing on understandings from Rogers' model, Biley (1992) has written about older people's sometimes different perceptions of time. She argues that, for some older people, time may seem to pass very slowly, and diversional therapies can be a useful aid to help to counteract long periods of inactivity. Using such techniques, the elderly woman may be helped to evoke memories of a happier time in her life. She may be encouraged to visualise pleasant things and people from her past to help to induce greater psychological awareness and a sense of self-worth and harmony.

During such interventions, the nurse will learn more about the woman's earlier life, and this will enable her to further repattern the environmental field with that of the woman. To do this, she might talk about things that were previously important for the woman and that relate to what they might be doing together. If she goes shopping with the woman, the nurse will be able to ask her about what she sees as important in window displays, for example.

The nurse may also discover what things amuse the woman and may be able to use these to promote laughter. Evidence for the therapeutic value of laughter is scarce, but both Malinski (1991) and Mallett (1995) point to its potential for achieving positive outcomes in terms of forgetting problems, reducing anxiety, feeling good and promoting hopefulness.

Evaluation

As acknowledged above, nowhere is Rogers' model more challenging than in trying to evaluate the degree of success achieved in repatterning someone's energy field. What is clear, however, is the necessity to focus evaluation on the whole person and not, for example, on body parts. Ference (1989) suggests evaluating a person's manifestations of his or her energy fields and also advocates assessing what she terms 'comfort levels'. Although her work focuses on the care of those who are dying, it may be that individuals' comfort with their situation could be a useful indicator of the successful repatterning of their energy field and a consequent decrease in dis-ease.

Such an outcome – the parents' greater comfort with, or acceptance of, their son's behaviour – might well signify successful intervention in the first example discussed here. If this is achieved, it may have positive effects on the little boy himself in both the short and the long term. In the short term, he may experience less dis-ease in his home enviroment, which may in turn temper his activity levels. Other changes to his environment, such as more muted decorative colours and a repatterning of his energy field through, for example, body massage, may also result in periods of increased rest and sleep. In the longer term, he stands to benefit from his parents' greater comfort with his uniqueness so that his behaviour is more accepted and labelled less as 'abnormal'.

For the woman who has recently moved into a residential home, the nurse is hoping to achieve a greater sense of peace and less anxiety in the new environment. She will therefore look for fewer verbal expressions of anxiety and loneliness from the woman and for less wandering in search of companionship. While a marked improvement in the woman's short-term memory remains unlikely, a greater comfort and ease within the new environment might be expected to lead to some improvement.

Two particular and important issues can be identified from the examples cited in this chapter. The first is that there may be times when gaining an understanding of the ideas encompassed in Rogers' model may be beneficial to those seeking health care as well as to the nurses providing that care. For the parents of the overactive boy, there is much to be gained from looking at a rather different explanation for his behaviour, one which no longer labels him 'abnormal'. Second, the need for nurses to be innovative in their intervention and evaluative strategies is paramount. From the examples cited here, there may be value in nurses developing tools to measure whole person comfort as a means of addressing some of the challenges posed by trying to evaluate care organised around Rogers' model.

References

Atherton, K. (1995) Homeopathy. In Rankin-Box, D. (ed.) *Complementary Therapies*. Edinburgh, Churchill Livingstone.

Balke, B., Anthony, J. and Wyatt, F. (1989) The effects of massage treatment on exercise fatigue. *Clinical Sports Medicine*, 1, 189–96.

Biley, F.C. (1992) The perception of time as a factor in Rogers' science of unitary human beings: a literature review. *Journal of Advanced Nursing*, 17, 1141–5.

Cowling, W.R. (1990) A template for nursing practice. In Barrett, E.A.M. (ed.) *Visions of Rogers' Science-Based Nursing*. New York, National League for Nursing.

Ference, H.M. (1989) Comforting the dying: nursing practice according to the Rogerian model. In Riehl-Sisca, J.P. (ed.) *Conceptual Models for Nursing Practice*. Norwalk, CT, Appleton & Lange.

Horrigan, C. (1995) Massage. In Rankin-Box, D. (ed.) *Complementary Therapies*. Edinburgh, Churchill Livingstone.

Krieger, D. (1979) *Therapeutic Touch: How To Use Your Hands To Help or Heal*. Englewood Cliffs, NJ, Prentice-Hall.

Krieger, D. (1981) *Foundations for Holistic Health Nursing Practices*. Philadelphia, J.B. Lippincott.

Longworth, J.C.D. (1982) Psychophysiological effects of slow stroke massage in normotensive females. *Advances in Nursing Science*, July, 44–6.

Lutjens, L.R.J. (1991) *Martha Rogers: The Science of Unitary Human Beings*. London, Sage.

Malinski, V.M. (1991) The experience of laughing at oneself in older couples. *Nursing Science Quarterly*, 4(2): 69–75.

Mallett, J. (1995) Humour and laughter therapy. In Rankin-Box, D. (ed.) *Complementary Therapies*. Edinburgh, Churchill Livingstone.

Mills, A. and Biley, F.C. (1994) A case study in Rogerian nursing. *Nursing Standard*, 9(7): 31–4.

Parker, K.P. (1989) The theory of sentience evolution: a practice level theory of sleeping, waking and beyond waking patterns based on the science of unitary human beings. *Rogerian Nursing Science News*, 2, 4–6.

Quinn, J.F. (1981) Client care and nurse involvement in a holistic framework. In Krieger, D. (ed.) *Foundations for Holistic Health Nursing Practices*. Philadelphia, J.B. Lippincott.

Rogers, M.E. (1970) *An Introduction to the Theoretical Basis of Nursing*. Philadelphia, F.A. Davies.

Rogers, M.E. (1980) Nursing: a science of unitary man. In Riehl, J.P. and Roy, C. (eds) *Conceptual Models for Nursing Practice*. Norwalk, CT, Appleton-Century-Crofts.

Rogers, M.E. (1983) Science of unitary human beings: a paradigm for nursing. In Clements, I. and Roberts, F. (eds) *Family Health: A Theoretical Approach to Nursing Care*. New York, John Wiley & Sons.

Rogers, M.E. (1989) Nursing: a science of unitary human beings. In Riehl-Sisca, J.P. (ed.) *Conceptual Models for Nursing Practice*, 3rd edn. Norwalk, CT, Appleton & Lange.

Rogers, M.E. (1992) Nursing science and the space age. *Nursing Science Quarterly*, 5, 27–34.

Sayre-Adams, J. (1995) Therapeutic touch. In Rankin-Box, D. (ed.) *Complementary Therapies*. Edinburgh, Churchill Livingstone.

Tomey, A.M. and Alligood, M.R. (1998) *Nursing Theorists and their Work*. St Louis, C.V. Mosby.

Afterword

Since we wrote the first edition of this book, *Nursing Models and the Nursing Process*, in the mid-1980s, the understanding of the contribution that models of nursing can make to patient care has developed enormously. Now, many more nurses are familiar with using a model to guide their practice, and this familiarity has enabled nurses to make informed decisions on the suitability of a particular model for the patients for whom they care.

In addition, nurses feel less uncertain about and constrained by the ideas incorporated in models. At one time, a nurse working with a particuar model tended to follow the nursing theorist's approach rather rigidly. Now, with greater confidence about the best ways in which to use models, nurses are able to be more innovative in developing care plans with patients while at the same time remaining true to the model's central concepts. This is a welcome advance in the application of models to nursing practice as it means that interventions can be better tailored to patients' needs.

As we enter the twenty-first century, nurses will be able to develop further their understanding of models and the frameworks for care that they offer. This will help nurses to respond appropriately to government initiatives that advocate greater professionalism in health care practitioners and that rely on a high-quality work force for their success. Nursing models go a long way towards enabling nurses to develop the unique body of knowledge essential for any profession. From such a body of knowledge, nurses will be in a position to extend the quality and effectiveness of their work still further.

It seems likely that current demands for increased partnership in health care will continue in the twenty-first century. Nurses working with nursing models will be in a stronger position to contribute on an equal footing with other health professionals so that those individuals with health-related problems, or who need health advice, can be assured of the best-quality service.

Index

Index

C

care
  disease-orientated approach 28
  individualisation of 19

care, key components of
  Henderson's model 31–6
  Johnson's model 63–6
  King's model 118–23
  medical model 27–30
  Neuman's model 150–4
  in nursing models 18
  Orem's model 97–104
  Peplau's model 134–9
  Riehl model 165–70
  Rogers' model 183–6
  Roper–Logan–Tierney model 46–51
  Roy adaptation model 79–85

care decisions, case example, King's
  model 123–32

care delivery
  Henderson's model 40–2
  Johnson's model 73–4
  King's model 130–1
  Orem's model 112–14
  Roper–Logan–Tierney model 57–9
  Roy adaptation model 92–4

care plan implementation, see
  intervention

care planning, see planning

case examples, see under individual
  models and subject headings

chemotherapy and body image
  changes, case example, Roy
  adaptation model 86–95

childbirth preparation, case example,
  Henderson's model 38–43

Chinese medicine 26, 181

'Cinderella' services 2–3

clinical effectiveness, information pack
  for self-evaluation of 10

clinical supervision 10

cognator subsystem, Roy adaptation
  model 81

comfort levels, Rogers' model 194

communication, King's model 119, 122

community psychiatric nursing, case
  example, Riehl model 170–9

complementarity (integrality) 184

complementary medicine 182–3

conceptual models of nursing, see
  nursing models

confronting stimuli, see focal stimuli

consent to treatment 4

contextual stimuli 80, 80–1, 85, 89

cultural differences, case example,
  Neuman's model 155–61

D

decision-making, by patients 4

defence, lines of, Neuman's model 150

delegation 11
  Henderson's model 41

dependent-care agency, Orem's model
  104, 107, 112, 113

dependent-care deficit, Orem's model
  97

depression 27–8

development model, see Peplau's
  development model

developmental self-care needs, Orem's
  model 99–100

developmental stages, human,
  Roper–Logan–Tierney model 48

diagnosis
  medical model 28
  see also nursing diagnosis

diaries, in health promotion 160

dis-ease alleviation, Rogers' model
  185, 187

Index

Index

Index

Index

Neuman's model 151, 154

student nurses, *see* nursing students

suicide attempt, case example 170–9

Sullivan's theory of human nature 134–6
dynamisms 135
euphoria 134
fundamental drives 134–5, 136
satisfaction drive 134, 135
security need 134, 135
tensions 134–5, 136
transformations 135

summative evaluation 16
Henderson's model 35, 43
Johnson's model 65–6
medical model 29
nursing process 21–2
Orem's model 116–17
Riehl model 179
Roper–Logan–Tierney model 51, 60–1
Roy adaptation model 95

supervision 10

survival factors, Neuman's model 150

sustenal imperatives, Johnson's model 65, 70, 73

symbolic interactionism 163, 164, 171–2

symbols, in communication 163–4

systems model of nursing, *see* Neuman's systems model

systems theory 78

T

tensions, in Sullivan's theory of human nature 134–5, 136

therapeutic self-care demand, Orem's model 100

Tierney, Alison 45

training, *see* education

transaction, King's model 119, 122

transformations, Sullivan's theory of human nature 135

U

unitary field model, *see* Rogers' unitary field model

unitary human fields, Rogers' model 183

United Kingdom Central Council for Nursing, Midwifery and Health Visiting (UKCC)
on advance directives 5
delegation guidelines 11

universal self-care needs, Orem's model 98–9

universe of open systems, Rogers' model 183

W

waiting lists 3

wellness, variation from, Neuman's model 152, 154, 155–7